G000123018

PLEASURE
CONSUMING
MEDICINE

SHETLAND LIBRARY
WITHDRAWN

91154708

PLEASURE

CONSUMING

MEDICINE

...

The Queer Politics
of Drugs

KANE RACE

Duke University Press
Durham & London
2009

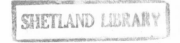
SHETLAND LIBRARY

© 2009 Duke University Press
All rights reserved
Printed in the United States
of America on acid-free paper ∞
Designed by Amy Ruth Buchanan
Typeset in Whitman by
Keystone Typesetting, Inc.
Library of Congress Cataloging-in-
Publication Data appear on the last
printed page of this book.

CONTENTS

...

PREFACE

. . .

A group called Freedom from Fear can serve as a brief illustration and entry point into the mutually transforming relations between medical subjectivity and consumer society that underlie and inform this book. It's one example of the patient advocacy and support groups that characterize the scene of health and medicine today. The group is a not-for-profit organization whose mission is to raise awareness about anxiety and depression and their treatment. Since its inception in 1984 it has become a national advocacy organization with many chapters and a significant media presence in the United States. A large amount of its funding comes from pharmaceutical organizations, which may help to explain its growth. The group promotes a range of drug and behavioral therapies and conducts awareness-raising activities, such as running the National Anxiety Disorders Freedom Day—a major media event. Here, medical education becomes indistinguishable from marketing, and health is thought to require consumer identification, as even the group's founder, Mary Guardino, advises: "One of the things I've found when you're reaching consumers is you have to have a good tag line. You have to give them a quick message that raises their curiosity and interest and says, 'Wow! That could be me!' "[1]

I first came across Freedom from Fear when Guardino was interviewed for *Selling Sickness*, a documentary that investigates the relations between medical science, the pharmaceutical industry, and contemporary society.[2] Couched in a genre that is increasingly well adapted to the intrigues of the contemporary pharmaceutical industry—detective journalism and exposé—the documentary forms part of a mounting critique of "disease-mongering."[3] This term was coined by a loose coalition of activists and medical professionals to describe the rapid expansion of disease categories driven by the profit motives of pharmaceutical corporations. While I don't wish to deny the importance of this effort to expose corporate interests and investigate their sociomedical effects, I did begin to wonder what would happen if we suspended its terms for just a moment and took initiatives such as Guardino's at face value for the insight they provide into the terms of medical rationality today. Guardino's commitment to her version of therapeutic salvation is evident in the film: she describes her personal experience at a promotional event where she suggests that, if all else fails, it is really worth trying an antidepressant. In another scene she is shown, perhaps gratuitously, recounting her story and exhorting her audience: "After I overcame all these things I said 'Why wouldn't anybody really want to take some drugs if it could help them to overcome their terrible life?' "

Well, precisely. The starting point for this book is the irony of a situation in which the medical industry persistently succeeds in widening the parameters of the uses to which drugs are put, while a punitive war on drugs escalates that takes a similar form of widening as its justification. I want to ask how, why, and with what effects contemporary strictures around the "improper" use of drugs are so ruthlessly maintained, while in the medical sphere the liberal application of drugs for varied purposes is increasingly promoted as a simple matter of consumer choice. In the current biomedical context, corporeal existence has become a privileged site for experiments with subjectivity.[4] This being the case, what purpose does the legal distinction between licit and illicit drugs serve, and why does it wield medical authority so selectively to demarcate the bounds of moral citizenship and identity? My aim in asking this question is not exactly to endorse a free market in drugs, for drugs do demand great care, but rather to use this perverse coincidence to open up a series of questions about how best to conceive the relations between drugs, bodies, subjectivities, identities, and practices. For if regulatory regimes determining the illicit use of drugs have acquired excessive power to frame individuals as normal or abnormal, decent or deviant—with criminal and damaging effects—as I will argue, then different conceptions and practices of responsibility—practices capable of attending more carefully to particular uses of drugs and relations of consumption—might have a better chance of preparing subjects for a society already permeated by drugs.

Initiatives such as Freedom from Fear embody many of the paradoxes, possibilities, and tough dilemmas of a situation I refer to in this book as "pleasure consuming medicine." This phrase aims to evoke the contemporary enthusiasm for drugs, in a deliberately ominous gesture. But it also tries, however improbably, to inject an element of hope and embodied inquiry into this situation—principally by activating the critical agency of pleasure. Pleasure is more or less absent from serious talk within public health, though it is a common enough motive for, and element of, human activity.[5] When it comes to drugs, it could be said to provide the basis upon which legal and moral distinctions (between licit and illicit instances) are made. Taking drugs for pleasure would appear to transgress the moral logic of "restoring health" that guarantees their pharmaceutical legitimacy. But the undeniable importance and common appeal of pleasure might lead us to wonder whether this routine exclusion and disavowal of pleasure doesn't serve to prop up the self-evidence of medical rationality. Enabling pleasure is one of medicine's most basic concerns, after all. Though the pursuit of pleasure is frequently projected onto others in efforts to expose them as intolerably indulgent— positioned as a vice pursued only by the marginal or depraved, or a luxury conceded only to the privileged—pleasure can be framed more generally as a need or aspiration that informs all manner of human activity. It has a generalizable or "whatever" quality that might also prompt a more expansive inquiry into particularity. Anyone can relate to the need for pleasure, though the precise content of what they are relating to may remain an open question. Against the blinking incomprehension that confronts unhealthy behavior, then, pointing to pleasure can function as a claim on understanding, an insistence on agency, and a sort of challenge. Situated in this way, pleasure offsets the actuarial calculation of risks and harms with a more situated inquiry into the terms of everyday life, while evoking a sense of agency and experimentation that the redemptive category of "self-medication" is unable to capture. No longer framed as restoring some natural order, drug use becomes intelligible as a specific intervention with specific consequences that is at any rate only one of a number of possible interventions.

Recent inquiries into pleasure provide an alternative vocabulary of experience than that propounded by the pharmaceuticalization of everyday life. Much of the recent work on affect seeks to value the sensibilities, pleasures, odd feelings, and attachments that are not immediately legible within a normative frame.[6] While consumer desires and expectations concerning pharmaceuticals are often conceived in terms of the commercial duping of consumers, they might be approached more comprehensively and understood as the product of wider norms around personhood, performance, health, and gender (for example), norms to which both patients and clinicians subscribe.[7] To the extent that some medications are prescribed on the basis of an apprehension of lived experience according to the reductive terms of *normal* and *abnormal*, *functional* and *dysfunctional*, it is possible that queer analysis, which historically has taken the social construction of normality as its object of critique, could offer important resources for grasping experience otherwise, in such a way as to withstand the more limiting implications and debilitating effects of drug regimes. One of the unfortunate effects of the narrative of disease-mongering, though, is that it discounts the experience of those who report specific value from pharmaceutical intervention. In its bid to protect the public from the corporate machinations of drug companies, this narrative ends up positing certain experiences of the body and subjects as "cultural dopes."[8] Crucial and timely as the critique of commercial influence may be, it finally doesn't know what to do with the consumer experience of drug regimes. It is as though the slur of commercial influence is enough to dismiss any subjective account of benefit from drugs as erroneous.

In contrast to this position, the present volume expresses no fundamental objection to people using drug technologies to address their situations. It simply argues that one frame that might viably inform such projects is that of pleasure, a word I use to evoke careful experimentation with the givenness of life, its materialities, conditions, contingencies, and specific relations. The book tries to open up a space, in other words, in which our engagements with potent substances could become intelligible outside of some of the more blatant pressures and inducements of normalization, and depend less for their authorization on adopting a prescriptive identity as sick.[9] This is not to deny the material requirements and physical predicaments of bodies. As will become clear in my discussion of HIV treatment in chapters 2 and 5, normative prescriptions surrounding medication use can themselves promote a certain degree of inattention to unwanted bodily events. Like it or not, drugs—both licit and illicit—are a significant part of contemporary practices of self-transformation, and the challenge is to reckon with the material effects of these intoxications in their multiplicity and complexity.

In the final pages of the first volume of *The History of Sexuality*, Foucault proposes "bodies and pleasures" as a potential rallying point against the regime of sexuality.[10] He contrasts bodies and pleasures with "sex and desire," whose insistent examination, he believes, will only bind us more tightly within this regime. The remarks are cryptic and under-developed and have been the source of some confusion. After all, Foucault spends most of the first volume detailing how bodily experience, sexual pleasure, and desire enter into the machinery of power and confession. Since he rejects the idea that power works simply by repressing personal desires and sexual pleasure, but rather demands their articulation and examination, it is initially unclear how an assertion of bodies and pleasures could resist the regime he describes. From a series of late interviews, it emerges that the key to understanding Foucault's proposal concerning bodies and pleasures relates to the distinction he makes between pleasure and desire in terms of their relation to expert knowledge.[11] Unlike desire, pleasure was not the object of an institutionalized theory; there was no science linking it to the nature of the human subject. Where psychoanalysis purported to offer a theory of desire, depicting its structures, and proposing it as a universal law that drives the human subject, pleasure remained relatively untheorized, and could not be used to diagnose individuals. Pleasure was less caught up in the whole apparatus that extracts a truth-value from embodied experience— all those therapeutic strategies whose diagnoses presuppose special insights into individuals on the basis of supposedly universal norms of desire. In this sense, pleasure could be regarded as much more open to historical construction, practical variation, and creative experimentation. It need not invoke some prediscursive domain of lived experience, as some have worried—it is social and historical material, through and through. It provided a way of approaching the forms of creative experimentation and world-building which were going on around Foucault in queer communities, with the added advantage of being relatively less encumbered by therapeutic or theoretical prescription.

Of course today, pleasure may not enjoy such luxury. Normative models of reward pathways riddle the popular and scientific literature on addiction, while as early as the 1940s, the concept of anhedonia (literally, the inability to feel pleasure) was being cited in American psychiatry in order to prescribe certain patients speed.[12] Nevertheless, there are good reasons for thinking that Foucault's take on pleasure as a social pragmatic may be useful for approaching some of the issues raised within contemporary drug regimes. Foucault's work on the history of sexuality was undertaken, not in any attempt to *know* sexuality, but rather to understand the forms of power that, in taking life as their object, subject people to disciplinary and normalizing regimes. In his subsequent work on "care of the self," he wanted to conceive forms of care and relation that could pry themselves away from normative determinations where necessary, but retain some form of ethical stylization.[13] I discuss the significance of this intervention for HIV/AIDS work in some detail in my final chapters. But to cut to the chase, Foucault's comments about bodies and pleasures indicate a preference for experimental practice over theory: he was interested in the cultures that marginalized groups were creating and their possibilities—including the possibility of creating innovative cultures of care. Grasped in this way, pleasure prompts a focus on what people actually do, rather than the nature of their desires; it directs attention to those material encrustations and innovations of practice that frequently escape or lay aside sovereign intention. For pleasure is expressive of a contradictory motion, in a sense that is significant for many of the activities considered in this book, in that it is capable of evoking, at once, the will and momentary excursions from the will.[14] To do as one pleases is not always to do as one expects.

Pleasure also references a body of work on the politics of consumption influenced by the Birmingham tradition of subcultural studies. Taking its distance from Frankfurt School pessimism (whose model of consumption it caricatured with the smacked-out figure of the cultural dope) this literature approaches consumption as a site of symbolic and creative play through which oppositional identities are forged.[15] Here, the consumer is depicted as actively involved in the creation and negotiation of consumption effects. Meaning is not fixed once and for all in consumer objects, but rather depends on the social practices in which their use is embedded. The question of how objects are taken up and used—how certain qualities are modified through enunciation—becomes a matter of investigation and a certain political longing. The Gramscian coordinates of this tradition frequently have the effect of reifying pleasure *as* resistance in a celebratory but hollow gesture. In the search for resistance, it unwittingly attributes an excess of agency and radical effect to the mere fact of consumer activity. But as I argue in this book, the more concrete sociology of "uses and pleasures" that is also found within this literature might lend health research much needed specificity. In the field of drug policy, for example, proponents of "harm reduction" work with the understanding that an appreciation of the different circumstances of drug use is crucial for averting harm: The effects of a drug can alter significantly depending on how, where and when it is used. Yet what becomes clear when adopting this approach is how it runs up against normative instatements of medicine. As I venture in chapters 2 and 3, the categories of drug abuse and noncompliance are alike in that they each describe any use of drugs that diverges from medical prescription as delinquent. In this moment, the capacity to distinguish between different practices of use is arrogated from above. Careful inquiry into the specificity of drug practices is disqualified in advance, in a move that divorces questions of drug use from embodied attention.

Of course, the hope of overcoming a terrible life is not the only reason someone might be inclined to take drugs. Pleasure is a common motive, and it enters as a key component into the making of moral and legal distinctions. But while this rationale is typically used to disqualify certain practices of drug use from moral comprehension, I contend that greater attentiveness to pleasure and its qualities and social dynamics may also provide crucial resources for devising more effective strategies of care. Though the present legal framework produces a drug culture that is shallow, individualistic, and criminal, I argue that mundane but consequential practices of safety, care, and differentiation still manage to circulate in this environment, where they form part of the recreational, ethical, or practical repertoire of participants in innumerable ordinary scenes and taste communities. I do not wish to deny the real harms, dangers, and devastation associated with some circumstances of drug use. But it becomes apparent that some fairly detailed strategies and technical vocabularies have emerged around the use of some illicit substances, from which there is something to learn. Such practices are fragile, and prone to being shamed out of existence. They are difficult to register in the current punitive political climate. In order to perceive them, it is necessary to consider pleasure, not as the antithesis of safety, but as the medium through which certain practices of safety take shape. For if drugs are now part of popular culture—a point that is difficult to dispute in the context of consumerized medicine—then it is to the vectors of popular culture—the dynamic exchanges of bodies, affects, values, tastes, and judgment—that we might turn if we are interested in promoting an intelligent public culture with respect to drug use.

ACKNOWLEDGMENTS

...

I have been fortunate to enjoy the guidance, support, and encouragement of many people over the course of this inquiry. The project initially took shape under the guidance of Rosalyn Diprose and Helen Keane, who have offered invaluable clarification, encouragement, and heartening comprehension of the concerns this book embodies throughout its many strange incarnations. I want to thank both of them for their wise advice and the inspiration of their work. The initial manuscript was written at the National Centre in HIV Social Research at the University of New South Wales, and I have my colleagues there to thank for teaching me what I know about social science, in particular Susan Kippax, whose interventions into HIV social research have been so crucial. Sue has expressed unwavering support for my work over many years, for which I am immensely grateful. From the field of HIV social research and public health, I have learnt a great deal from discussions with John Ballard, Colin Batrouney, Jonathan Bollen, Alan Brotherton, June Crawford, Simon Donohoe, Ross Duffin, Jeanne Ellard, Maude Frances, Suzanne Fraser, Martin Holt, Michael Hurley, John Imrie, Phillip Keen, Julie Letts, David McInnes, Dean Murphy, Christy Newman, Marcus O'Donnell, Asha Persson, Patrick Rawstorne, Edward Reis, Sean Slavin, Gary Smith, kylie valentine, Paul Van de Ven, Russell Westacott, Heather Worth, and many others. Among colleagues at the University of New South Wales, Catherine Mills, Nicholas Rasmussen, Catherine Waldby, and Elizabeth Wilson engaged me in thought-provoking discussions around medicine, pharmaceuticals, and society. Students in my course "Bodies, Habits, and Pleasures" provided a lively context for further thought and work. Thanks must go to Kath Albury and Tobin Saunders for putting on a good show, and to Brent Beadle for suggesting I watch it. I am grateful to Carol Boyd, Joseph Jewitt, Elspeth Probyn, Robert Reynolds, Elizabeth Wilson, and

Heather Worth for the opportunities they provided to present parts of this research. Moira Gatens, Paul Morrison, Cindy Patton, Elspeth Probyn, and anonymous readers from Duke University Press made generous and incisive readings of different versions of this manuscript, and I thank them for their suggestions. Thanks in particular to my editor at Duke University Press, Ken Wissoker, for his good advice, confidence in this project, and patience.

The final manuscript of this book was prepared largely over the course of a Visiting Fellowship at the Institute for Research on Women and Gender at the University of Michigan in 2007, which in turn was made possible through a period of study leave generously granted to me by the Department of Gender and Cultural Studies at the University of Sydney. I can't imagine having completed this book without this opportunity, or without access to the intellectual climate afforded to me by new colleagues and friends, and I would like to thank both institutions for enabling this period of work. Thanks to the staff and students at the University of Sydney, especially Jane Park, Elspeth Probyn, and Catherine Driscoll, for welcoming me into the Department of Gender and Cultural Studies. I would also like to thank Barry Adam, Carol Boyd, Marcy Epstein, Paul Farber, Robbie Griswold, Pascal Grosse, Alejandro Herrero-Olaizola, Renee Hoogland, Trevor Hoppe, Jonathan Metzl, Michele Morales, Jack Tocco, Gregory Tomso, Russell Westhaver, and Susan Wright for the friendship and encouragement they provided while I was at the University of Michigan, and for their responses to this work as it developed. Spending time with Ross Chambers, who offered encouragement, good company, and extensive feedback on some sections, was a real delight. David Caron never failed to inspire me with his friendship, tact, strategic tactlessness, and general engagement with the world. Thanks also to Jeff and Paul.

I thank the editors and publishers of the following journals for allowing me to include revised versions of earlier articles as part of this book: "The Death of the Dance Party," *The Australian Humanities Review* 30 (October 2003), http://www.australianhumanitiesreview.org; "Drugs and Domesticity: Fencing the Nation," *Cultural Studies Review* 10, no. 2 (2004): 62–84; "Recreational States: Drugs and the Sovereignty of Consumption," *Culture Machine* 7 (2005), http://www.culturemachine.net; "The Undetectable Crisis: Changing Technologies of Risk," *Sexualities* 4, no. 2 (2001): 167–89. I also thank Johns Hopkins University Press, the National Association of People with AIDS in Australia, and John Spooner and the *Age* newspaper for allowing me to reproduce images produced or held by them, the sources of which are acknowledged in further detail within.

David, Susan, and Cleo Race supported this project unconditionally despite its unfamiliar nature and aspirations, inspiring my respect and deep gratitude as well as love. Thanks also to Nic Frankham, Cath Le Couteur, Brent Mackie, John Sinatore, Aldo Spina, Joanne Thorley, and Richard Williamson for sustaining me and laughing with me over the course of this project. Five people have offered particularly important contexts for friendship, intellectual exchange, and inspiration to me over this period. Marsha Rosengarten has been a generous interlocutor and cothinker around questions of HIV, medicine, and critical scholarship for many years. Niamh Stephenson has similarly helped me think through innumerable questions around medical and social experience. Many pleasurable moments in the writing of this book stem from working with Gay Hawkins, a wonderful thinker, writer, colleague, and teacher. And I especially want to thank David Halperin, who has been a vital source of encouragement, intellectual sustenance, and practical inspiration over the course of this project, and ever since. Without these colleagues, this work would have been a far less pleasurable and probably impossible adventure. My heartfelt thanks, finally, to Adrian Kerr, for his love, his tenderness, and the life we share—it's to him that I dedicate this work.

Curiosity . . . evokes "care"; it evokes the care one takes of what exists and what might exist; a sharpened sense of reality, but one that is never immobilized before it; a readiness to find what surrounds us strange and odd; a certain determination to throw off familiar ways of thought and to look at the same things in a different way; a passion for seizing what is happening now and what is disappearing; a lack of respect for the traditional hierarchies of what is important and fundamental.

MICHEL FOUCAULT,

"The Masked Philosopher"

The drug-tinged adjectives "curious" and "subtle" [share] a built-in epistemological indecision or doubling. Each of them can describe, as the *OED* puts it, "an object of interest" . . . and, in almost the same terms, the quality of the perception brought by the attentive subject to such an object: for "curious" "as a subjective quality of persons," the *OED* lists, e.g., "careful, attentive, anxious, cautious, inquisitive, prying, subtle." The thing known is a reflection of the impulse towards knowing it, then, and each describable only as the excess, "wrought" intensiveness of that knowledge-situation.

EVE KOSOFSKY SEDGWICK,

Epistemology of the Closet

1

PLEASURE CONSUMING MEDICINE

• • •

An Introduction

My drugs require me to dance with no fewer
than ten thousand people at a time.
DAVID HALPERIN

This book explores multiple declensions of three seemingly incompatible terms: *pleasure, consuming,* and *medicine.* At first glance, "pleasure consuming medicine" is a queer conjunction. It doesn't seem to refer to any obviously recognizable form of experience. It is difficult to discern what it might properly mean. We are far more likely to consider medicine a bitter pill to swallow. Indeed, the austere advice to stop eating rich foods, exercise more, keep out of the sun, or give up smoking could well support the impression that medicine and pleasure are antithetically opposed. It is rare, in the presence of such advice, for pleasure to be treated as a valid exception to the medical rule. It tends to be cast instead as a gratuitous enticement that the individual must overcome in a dutiful struggle for health and self-mastery. From this perspective—and in ways that range from mildly irritating to thoroughly devastating—the imperatives of medicine can seem entirely pleasure-consuming.

Perhaps this loggerhead relation of medicine and pleasure has been felt most acutely in our time in the context of the AIDS crisis. Abruptly, many found their most intimate, exciting, or otherwise meaningful practices on the wrong side of (frequently punitive and distorted) health edicts. But while one very common response to this crisis might be summed up in the phrase "where safety prevails, pleasure must submit," HIV education has in fact been most effective when it has foregrounded and incorporated the embodied pleasures of endangered groups. The history of HIV prevention may be understood as a series of struggles on the part of affected groups to elaborate bodily practices capable of mediating between pleasure and safety. Here, health does not stand in opposition to pleasure. Rather it is something that has to be collaboratively negotiated and produced through the careful interaction of bodies. What can be drawn from this history is a better understanding of the critical agency of pleasure when devising practical logics of care and safety.

In general terms, though, the proposition that one might actually experience pleasure while consuming medicine seems slightly absurd. Indeed, it's easy to arrive at the conclusion that pleasure is precisely what should *not* be had in such activity. It is as though the two terms act, or should act, to cancel each other out. The clinician warns "this may feel a little uncomfortable" before engaging in procedures that can actually produce some not-entirely-unpleasant sensations. To acknowledge pleasure here would seem to betray the self that medicine must contain in its effort to produce a properly objective body, so pleasure is performatively banished from the clinic.[1] Likewise, medical procedures are routinely demarcated from the realm of aesthetics. Reconstructive surgery is distinguished from cosmetic surgery, for example, on the basis of medical need and with reference to structures of the body that are classed as abnormal (in need of repair) rather than normal (and desiring adornment).[2] In each of these instances, it seems important that health be not contaminated by more specific modes of desire—that it be basic, unmarked, and devoid of any affective connotation. To introduce particular affects into these contexts would be to excise health from medicine's recuperative function. Medicine concerns itself with the grave task of restoring life to its proper order. It is not, first and foremost, about optimizing particular attributes and sensations. Of course, pleasure might be experienced as a corollary of restoring health. One could even be excused for feeling good at such a prospect. But taking medicine for pleasure, without the intermediary goal of restoring health in all its generality? Such a qualified and instrumental reassignment of medical priorities and values would initially seem impossible to admit.

What are we to make then of the popularity of a class of medicines whose utility can well be framed in terms of enhancement, rather than merely treatment?[3] In *Listening to Prozac*, psychiatrist Peter Kramer uses the term *cosmetic pyschopharmacology* to describe the sort of clinical and biochemical mechanisms at work in some applications of the antidepres-

sant fluoxetine.[4] Though initially his description frames the transformations enabled by this drug as superficial ("a neurochemical nosejob") and
even socially dangerous ("steroids for the business Olympics"),[5] Kramer
demonstrates in the course of his discussion the far-from-trivial ways in
which they can also transfigure the suffering of some patients. His account transfers clinical labor from a paradigm of restoration to one of
transformation. Out of his careful discussion of numerous case studies, a
picture of efficacy emerges that is not so much one of returning patients
to a prior or extraneous state of normality, but rather one in which
medicine produces quite specific sets of modifications to mood and
behavior, with both beneficial and adverse effects. The effects can be—
and in many cases are—critically evaluated in new forms of relation
between clinician, patient, and their associates. Kramer displays some
caution in characterizing medicine in these terms, but his book stands as
an intelligent account of how biochemistry is being enfolded, through
drugs, in new practices of ethical self-formation.

The tensions between treatment and enhancement play out particularly passionately in the case of a series of drugs that have acquired the
nickname "lifestyle drugs." The term encompasses medications aimed at
reversing baldness and losing weight as well as some applications of this
class of antidepressants, such as reducing inhibition and shyness. But it
inspires a particular level of excitement when it comes to drugs that
target matters sexual. Strains begin to show, it seems, when the pathological imagination is applied to a domain so firmly identified with pleasure.
In an article published in the *British Medical Journal* in 2003, Ray Moynihan reported on recent initiatives to clarify a category of female pathology.[6] Keen to reproduce the massive profits of Viagra, drug companies
were revealed to be sponsoring meetings between researchers and the
pharmaceutical industry to determine the definition and measurable
characteristics of "female sexual dysfunction" (FSD) as required for cred-
ible clinical trials. Data were being gathered to determine the "normal
physiologic responses" for women in particular age groups. "The corporate sponsored creation of a disease is not a new phenomenon," Moynihan wrote, "but the making of female sexual dysfunction is the freshest,
clearest example we have."[7] The article provoked a flurry of responses,
both for and against.[8] For some, FSD was a genuine disorder, a pathology
that feminists everywhere had a duty to affirm. To get the condition

recognized and achieve equality in the field of pharmaceutical production, women had to cast their claims in the language of essential pathology: women's sexuality *really can* be impeded by physiological deficiencies. The fight for recognition required a proliferation of testimony on the realness of the condition: moving accounts of the plight of those with the disorder, anger and resentment that the validity of women's claims was once again being put in question. To achieve a just outcome, the normative determinations of medicine were to be affirmed, and the inventive character of its taxonomic labor denied.[9] For others, though, FSD was "nothing more than a figment of corporate America's financial imagination," as Shere Hite put it, a cynical ploy of greedy multinationals bent on colonizing everyday life with biomedical artifacts and categories. FSD was not a "real" disease but a "construction"—a fact made all the more sinister by the involvement of industry. Hite, for example, complained that the pharmaceutical industry had "wilfully misunderstood the basics of female sexuality in its lust for blockbuster drugs."[10] In their bid to sell product to gullible consumers, the makers of "female Viagra" were imposing an individualizing and masculinist frame on female sexuality. In so doing, they were selling women the fantasy that the interpersonal, social, and material problems affecting women's lives and sexualities could be resolved by taking a pill. Not only was FSD based on a normative conception of female sexuality, obviating as a consequence the cultural and performative differences in this sphere; but once it was in circulation, it would also set new universalizing standards, reducing women's experience to the humiliating and coercive terms of functionality and dysfunction.

Without entering into a detailed discussion of this example, it seems necessary to insist that yes, there *is* a physiological dimension to a realm of experience known as sexuality—a realm whose existence must be acknowledged in the case of women as well as men—and yes, medical categories *are* constructed and arise out of a questionable blend of scientific and commercial resources, a blend whose concrete manifestations require critical attention. It is not enough, for example, to claim that because this category of disorder is constructed, it is therefore false—unless one is willing to posit some pure and preconstructed realm of actual experience. It is telling in this regard that it falls on female sexuality to provide the "freshest, clearest example" of the artificial machinations of capitalist medicine. Women's sexuality is thereby constructed as pure, natural, and essentially nonexistent—something that reveals more about the traditional status of female sexuality than any of the ethical implications of this instance. To claim, on the other hand, that this pathology is real, plain and simple—as some proponents do—is to ignore the consequential nature of scientific and epistemological production: the impact of its practices, its constitutive effects. How quickly the argument congeals into a rhetorical division between a realm of experience that is supposedly real, natural, and therefore needs to be constantly reaffirmed as the single and incontestable standard of experience and value, and the view that what is constructed is artificial, and thus duplicitous (a set of assignments whose unsettling character seems almost entirely pre-validated in existing suspicions surrounding the category "drug"). Yet what this example must reveal most powerfully is the enormous discursive and scientific labor, both within and outside medicine, that goes into characterizing the purpose of medicine *neutrally* (in terms of repairing disorder) rather than *positively* (as enhancement). Assuming the drug in development does have some tangible and even desirable effects for some, irrespective of pathology, what this example reveals quite clearly is how intent medical morality is on disavowing its own active involvement in creation and re-creation.

"Viagra is a recreational drug," writes Germaine Greer. "Ask the gay guys who keep Trade's club floor jumping and fill the pages of Attitude. They should know—they've been using it for months. And health is the least of their concerns. In hyper-gay circles, it is getting difficult to steer clear of Viagra. Any guy who would prefer to walk and talk, wine and dine, cuddle and kiss his significant other rather than keep him impaled for 48 hours is a sissy. When you can have a whole weekend of synthetic priapism, what red-blooded male would settle for anything less? Viagra weekends could vanquish football as we know it."[11] The concern over lifestyle drugs arises, in part, from a concern over public subsidization. Those aiming for subsidization must cast their claims in the language of essential injury and its repair, while opponents use the tag of "lifestyle" or "recreation" in order to dismiss the drug in question as trivial, its effects indulgent and, in the final instance, expendable. This is why Greer wants to characterize Viagra as recreational. Concerned about the state of care for "women, children, the elderly and the actually sick," she wants to question, in the case of erectile difficulty, the purchase that the medical determination of disorder has on the public imagination. One need not disagree with Greer's priorities here to query the terms she uses to make her argument. Viagra is coded as recreational by associating it with gay life, located squarely in the zones of leisure. This in turn works to separate out a domain of "necessity" from a domain marked "lifestyle," and the distinction gets mapped onto lives and identities in culturally consequential ways.[12] While some grading of need is unavoidable when it comes to the allocation of public resources for medical interventions, the way Greer deploys this distinction illustrates why the sexually minoritized have good reason to be suspicious of its cultural overtones. The distinction bears traces of gay men's already ambiguous status in the public sphere proper. Thus when, at a meeting on global treatment access, a pharmaceutical company representative responds to a demand made by AIDS activist Mark Harrington by asking, "Do you want us to leave the field and just work on lifestyle drugs?" I can't help reading this threat as, unconsciously or not, double-barrelled.[13]

One of the issues here is that the medical construction of pathology cannot be relied upon to provide an infallible guide to public, let alone global, need. This is why terms like "lifestyle" pop up repeatedly in the pharmaceutical domain: they attempt to patch over the gap between medical and state or insurer determinations of what counts as necessary repair. The capitalization of the life sciences has meant that the logic of financial returns and market share now dominates which products get developed.[14] As well as indicating a situation of massive geopolitical disparity—in which research and development for the major diseases affecting the world's poor is left languishing while minor problems that are expected to attract large financial returns are pursued[15]—this situation exposes a peculiarity of the contemporary medical gaze: the attribution of disorder cannot be regarded as an accurate measure of social or collective need, but references a generic body, extracted from any relational context, to whom the category of need can be infinitely and arbitrarily applied so long as there is the desire, prospect, and normative precedent for some form of enhancement. If the image of medicine cataloguing norms of everyday pleasure in order to authorize the development of marketable product evokes a more disturbing sense of pleasure consuming medicine, it also crystallizes a problem in the sphere of regulation. Because authorizing new drugs demands the endorsement of new pathologies, the only thing medicine may produce, in this discourse, is a return to a putative state of normality. But what is also reproduced in this move is the regulative power of medicine to determine what can count as normal and therefore properly and publicly desirable.

This raises the question of the organizing power of the cultural classification of drugs. In 1982, a World Health Organization memorandum defined *drugs* (the illicit sort) as "any chemical entity or mixture of entities, other than those required for the maintenance of normal health, the administration of which alters biological function and possibly structure."[16] As Olmo writes, "Despite being imprecise and overly generalized, this definition has been repeated ad infinitum in scores of specialized texts in diverse countries, without further elaboration."[17] Here, "normal health" appears as an exit clause that redeems certain chemical modifications of the body, while the presence of any purpose outside this ambit condemns the use in question to illegitimacy. This definition allows drugs and their classification to compose a site at which abnormal and normal functions of the body are revealed. Thus in one article gay "habitués of the circuit" are described as using "one kind of drug to heighten their sexual energies and another to relax their sphincter muscles."[18] Such activities incur a disapproval that is usually reserved for the chemical substances themselves, accentuating the misuse of organs already presumed to be implicit in homosexuality, redoubling these activities as synthetic and dangerous pursuits. For Greer, too, a sense of the proper function of the male body, represented in heterosexual conjugal sex, informs her understanding of the proper function of Viagra, with uses falling outside this ambit considered recreational. Thus, though great pains have been taken by authorities to portray the inability to get an erection on demand as a debilitating ailment, this taxonomy of need is quickly undone when the focus shifts to how the product is actually used.[19]

Another short illustration of some of the practical impasses of the cultural logic of treatment occurs in the case of those very essential (but, for much of the world's infected population, still largely inaccessible) drugs that work to reduce the rate of HIV viral replication in the body. Though these medicines were initially celebrated as bringing a form of closure to the HIV epidemic, it soon became apparent among those with some experience of them that a straightforward return to normality was an inadequate way of characterizing their biochemical and cultural activity. The treatments became associated with a range of harmful physical effects including diarrhea, nausea, high blood pressure, liver damage, insomnia, fatigue, hallucinations, depression, memory problems, and other unknown and perhaps irreversible dangers. Perhaps most unexpected and distressing for many was a metabolic disorder known as lipodystrophy, which comprises an accumulation of fat in some parts of the body combined with wasting of the face, arms, legs, and buttocks.[20] This concern was first identified in (and frequently downplayed as a function of) gay urban cultures in which body-consciousness is highly valued. When patients complained about these effects, for example, their concern was sometimes characterized by clinicians, whose goal was to promote treatment compliance, as "cosmetic"—a mere function of lifestyle—which had the effect of trivializing the materiality of these cultural norms.[21] At the same time, medical researchers were working to codify the characteristics of this experience with the aim of legitimating it as an objective medical condition—a process that required them to smooth over the mutual contingency of treatment and culture. At the time of writing, advocates for people living with HIV were facing this discursive quandary again as they pushed for a trial of a product called New-Fil, which conceals the signs of wasting to the face caused by the specific activity of HIV treatment. If this intervention is to be publicly subsidized (and thus accessible to those who would most benefit from it), advocates must frame it as a reconstructive rather than a cosmetic procedure. But this premium on "restoration" additionally covers over the iatrogenic character of medical intervention.

One aspect of the predicament is the exclusive equation of medical disorder with essential need, a problem that, as we have seen, is currently addressed by quarantining a realm called "lifestyle" from another, deemed "normal health," conceived as somehow not styled, but essential. But can this distinction really adequately frame what is being contested here? The solution is limited if it is applied in any preordained way. This is the problem that Greer faces in her claim that Viagra is recreational: she ends up reinstating a privileged zone of normality. But Greer is right—Viagra *is* recreational: it recreates the normative rigidity of penetrative penile sex. And it is in this sense that *all* medicines could be considered re-creational: they are involved in what Michael Hardt and Antonio Negri describe as the "continuous constituent project to create and re-create ourselves and our world."[22] They participate, that is to say, in the always risky and consequential process of making our nature—and in ways that constantly exceed the cultural logic of "cure." What medical drugs must be made to reveal, in other words, is the artifice—and political decision—involved even in the production of "normal" bodies.

When medicines are conceived in the supposedly benign terms of restoring an essential nature, their *surplus effects* recede from view. And when they are constituted merely as repair, their standardizing pressure materializes all the more forcefully. Thus one way to grasp the responsibility of drugs would be to consider them as *necessarily re-creational*. When all drugs are cast on the plane of re-creation, the agonistic nature of pharmaceutical production and consumption becomes explicit: we expose what is specific, partial, *and* consequential about our biochemical techniques of the self. The question (necessarily a political one) that emerges from such a conceptual re-signification is this: what are the forms of re-creation in which we—individually, collectively, corporeally—are to invest?[23]

Drug Regimes—A User's Guide

It is difficult to think through the tenuous nature of present freedoms within first world economies, but one would do well to link it to the sense of moral conformity that appears as an enthusiastic adjunct to consumerism in the citizen equation. While we are presented with endless depictions of peripheral pleasure, a rabid moralism obtains. As the political centers of imperial economies peel away the responsibilities of the welfare state, a recurring feature has been the investment of figures such as the *family*, *community*, and *nation* as moral buttresses whose task it is to safeguard decency and welfare. As governments shed their material functions, these figures take up the symbolic slack, enjoying their capacity to rally enthusiastic support from both ends of the political spectrum. The homogeneity these figures are intended to secure—the particular exclusions and privations they are proposed to effect—are less often remarked, because their presence is such a staple feature of every-day discourse: they are widely relied upon to offer comfort and security in contexts where these feelings are scarce. Meanwhile, it is rare that the rights and freedoms of sexual minorities, for example, are formally reversed. Instead, when politically expedient, moral panics about the threat of their difference are orchestrated. In this context, citizenship is redefined "through consumerism tied to moral conformity," formalizing degrees of citizenship according to categories of difference.[24] Thus, while minoritized subjects ostensibly enjoy many of the same civil rights as others—configured in terms of access to commodities and regard for privacy—the sense of "degrees of citizenship" and the threat of moral panic produce a tendency within these ranks to emulate the moral status of the mainstream, one tied to family—or, failing that, to the "shared values" of community. Meanwhile, the lately visible pleasures of different styles of life are consigned to the recreational sphere, where they are spectacularly available to be figured as superfluous.

These dynamics call for an analysis capable of contesting the uneven production of material reality, but in a manner that is careful not to consign the politics of bodies to a secondary or superfluous status. If the consumer context has enabled changes—some of them positive—to the conditions of access to public representation, it is nonetheless necessary to register the profound ambivalence of the liberties of market society: to dispute the whitewashing of alternate histories and futures by discourses of consumer choice. It is with this purpose in mind that I turn to drugs, not simply in despair, but with a view to understanding the forms of tweaking that have been adopted to finesse the present moment of globalization. Because drug consumption "tends to reproduce the conditions of destruction, not production," to borrow Andrew Ross's formulation, it poses a distinct challenge to those versions of liberal politics prone to overlooking the material inequities of bodies.[25] But, as readings of various drug texts show, these inequities are nonetheless discursively produced. As well as featuring at large in recent moral panics concerning sexuality and race, drug discourses reveal much about how bodies are geared up in the present of the global market, which bodies are prescribed and which abandoned. If globalization purportedly dismantles many of the constraints of the nation-state, drugs control stands out as a striking example of the ruthless ways in which the machineries of citizenship, its borders and controls, are clamped back down, in a sort of imperial insistence on the nation's contours and forms. As I will argue, drugs are fit for incorporation within an amoral consumer logic, as commodities par excellence, such that one is tempted to rephrase Michel Foucault's remarks about sex: Do not think that by saying yes to drugs, one is saying no to power. Yet, as illustrated in the actions of Australia's former prime minister John Howard—who intervened in the production of a national drug education resource so that it would bear the title "Our Strongest Weapon Against Drugs . . . Families"[26]—the forces that are marshalled to the cause of Just Say No reveal much about the broader strategies of political, economic, and bodily containment within economic liberalism.

It's a balmy summer night in 2007, and partygoers are making their way through the gardens at Lady Macquarie's Chair to attend the Azure Party on the harbor foreshore, an annual fixture of the gay and lesbian Mardi Gras. The Sydney Opera House gleams softly in the background, as though strategically positioned to court the global gay visitor. Planning for the party, as usual, has been extensive. Alongside the outfits, suntans, drugs, lights, DJs, and show preparations, parties like this are always closely monitored by health professionals and volunteers trained to deal with the occasional emergencies that are known to occur, and a volunteer care team of this sort has assembled. But with a state election around the corner, this event attracts an unanticipated form of attention, which, it could be said, creates an emergency of its own. Uniformed and plainclothes police officers are patrolling the gates with dogs trained to sniff out amphetamines, cannabis, cocaine, and other illegal substances. Mild panic ensues. Some patrons down all their drugs at once in an attempt to avoid detection, unable to face the prospect of wasting the dollars they had spent but putting themselves at heightened risk of danger and overdose. Others try their luck at the gates, hoping to evade the public humiliation of being searched and the possibility of a criminal record. Police with dogs roam around inside the party, apprehending individuals. By 9:00 p.m., twenty-six patrons are arrested with small quantities of illicit substances. At this point, a court order is obtained to shut down the party, and the remaining frazzled partygoers are dispersed into the Saturday night city streets.

This scene of intervention and panic expresses certain tensions within the government of drugs—tensions that lend themselves to a broader analysis of the political administration of consumer society and its strategic citation of biopolitical prerogatives. It's a scene whose casual violence is, if not already normalized, then rapidly becoming so, at youth events, in migrant, indigenous, and racially marked precincts, and in public, recreational, and transitional spaces in Western and "Westernizing" nations.[27] What is interesting is how the status of certain substances as "illicit" provides an occasion for the state to engage in what can be described as a disciplinary performance of moral sovereignty. This performance bears little relation to the actual dangers of drug consumption—in fact it exacerbates them, as we shall see. It is an exercise in the politics of *sending a message*, the ideological content of which bears further speculation. The illicit drug user has become a special and symbolic figure for the neoliberal state. These consumptive practices mirror the licensed pleasures of the market, but can also be made to exemplify their excess. When its authority or capacity to govern well is in question, the neoliberal state jumps at the chance to dramatize the ostensible danger of those pleasures that evade authoritative control. This makes unauthorized pleasure, rather than systemic factors or governmental practices, explain the broader experience and apprehension of danger and insecurity. Lauren Berlant uses the phrase "the intimate public sphere" to describe the ideological state in which personal acts—acts not necessarily directed toward the civic sphere, like sex—acquire a luminous power to "send a message" about the moral constituency of the nation and the conditions of belonging in it.[28] The drug test is the latest technology in this arsenal of power, and in the present climate of expanded consumer freedoms and identities, it is used to effect some of the same forms of privatization and individualization that queer theorists have identified in relation to sexuality.[29] Drugs would appear to encapsulate the risks of postmodern consumption for a nationalist and individualist imaginary that seeks to deflect social responsibility for current injustices by projecting, as counter to drugs, reified images of authenticity, familiarity, and individual morality (see chapter 4). In a context where citizenship is increasingly figured around the pleasures of consumption, drug use has emerged as a trope through which different relations to pleasure, consumption, embodiment, and medical authority are sensationalized.

The drug search cites the protection of the health of the population as its rationale, and, to be sure, the substances it targets are not without their dangers. This is why volunteer teams go to great lengths to devise care practices uniquely adapted to this environment, designed to respond quickly and effectively to possible emergencies. It is also why many drug users themselves devise fairly sophisticated dosing practices and routines, which aim—as far as possible within given constraints—to prevent adverse events.[30] Such care practices are made precarious by these practices of enforcement, and understanding this relation is one of the key aims of this book.[31] For in fact, the liberal state allows many forms of dangerous recreation, like football, mountain climbing, and drinking—experiences which, though dangerous, can also be fun and even profound.[32] One would be horrified if the state tried to make these legitimized forms of risk-taking as dangerous as possible in order to discourage people from trying them. But such is exactly what is allowed in the case of drug operations, which in their present form preclude quality control and threaten users.

The search at the Azure Party in 2007 followed the death of a young woman after her attendance at a youth music festival the previous week. The woman had taken a pill she believed to be ecstasy, but which was actually contaminated with PMA (paramethoxyamphetamine), a synthetic hallucinogen that can be lethal at high doses. Her death would appear to confirm the admonitions of public health posters plastered around Sydney at about this time, which advised, "There is no such thing as a standard pill." But this message only obscures the sense in which power gives rise to the very risks it warns against, by making quality control impossible and the content of illicit substances unreliable. Such obfuscation was carried over into the police handling of the woman's death. Police initially refused to release any identifying features of the pill associated with the death with a view to *sending a message* about the moral dangers of drug use. Thus, rather than give consumers practical information that might help to prevent further deaths, the prerogatives of health were subjugated, in typical fashion, to symbolic politics.

As a means of drug control, meanwhile, the use of drug detection dogs has been shown to be spectacularly unsuccessful. It uncovers drugs in only about a quarter of prompted searches, leading to successful convictions for drug supply in only the tiniest proportion of cases.[33] And the targeting of drug use in public space generates even riskier practices of consumption as users attempt to avoid detection. The long-term effect is to drive drug use underground, producing unprecedented challenges for health specialists by generating new, more covert, and more dangerous practices of consumption.[34] The persistence of these policing practices, despite their documented failures, raises questions, such as, why is the state prepared to override its biopolitical commitments *at the very moment* that it cites those biopolitical commitments most insistently? The contradictory effects of such operations and their ramification of entrenched patterns of social violence are not lost on those who are subject to them. Interviewed later by the *Sydney Morning Herald*, one Azure partygoer put it plainly: "I find it hard to believe the NSW Police shut down the party for the concern and health of the people at the party. If there was genuine concern from the police for partygoers then to me it would make sense to make an announcement to patrons and step up crowd monitoring. Instead, they ejected 5,000 people out of what was a medically supervised and policed event onto the streets to fend for themselves."[35]

The drug raid seizes upon and intercepts deviant groups and liminal practices, but, cloaking itself in the generality of drug law, claims not to target them specifically. This pretence makes such operations difficult to dispute through established channels, since the platform of minority identity that supports liberal criticisms of discriminatory treatment seems to dissipate in the face of the universal construction of the law. It's always possible, for example, for authorities to point to another operation where the minority in question was not the target. Thus, "objective" proscriptions concerning the possession of illicit substances are used forcibly to expose and confirm suspected categories of deviance in a maneuver that is pure spectacle, made for the headlines. What is striking about this operation is its use of a *technology of exposure* to conjure the moral state.[36] Indeed, the persistence of these policing practices despite the evidence accumulated against them suggests that their counterproductivity is beside the point. For the point is the public spectacle of detection and humiliation, the making suspect of populations, the performance of moral sovereignty and the opportunistic exposure of those who are deemed to have failed it. In periods of political instability and social unrest, the drug raid converts generalized insecurity into a matter of personal and moral regimes.

This book takes the drug search as emblematic of a broader technology of power that converges on embodiment, consumption, and pleasure in the name of health, while considering some of the spontaneous forms of resistance that have emerged in response. Two discourses associated with notions of the proper use of drugs have become particularly available for demarcating citizenship and revealing moral personhood in neoliberal societies: the medical discourse of patient compliance and the legal discourse of drug misuse or drug abuse. The discourse of compliance constructs a category of normal behavior around the extent to which patients' behavior coincides with clinical prescriptions. The discourse of drug abuse repeats this configuration of individual responsibility and deviance with respect to drugs in the law. Both these discourses took shape in the 1970s, just as economically liberal and socially conservative policies and ideas coalesced to produce the New Right. And they mirror each other in the sense that both take *self-administration* as their problem and object of concern, and both propose medicine as the proper authority against which to reference this conduct. The convergence of these discourses newly articulates the self at the intersection of health and consumption. At the moment that consumption becomes the normative mode of social participation and citizenship, medical authority becomes available in these discourses to fulfill the role of the moral curb on the self-administering consumer. As a result, these discourses become especially prone to political and authoritarian investment—precisely because they produce the *self* as the moral locus of consumption.

The general context of my analysis is the ideological investment in the "self" that has marked the shift from welfarist to neoliberal politics. But rather than focus directly on the implications of this shift for health care, as recent volumes have done,[37] my interest is in how health discourses—and particularly discourses on the proper use of drugs—have offered a ground for the ideological *performance* of this shift. Where Foucault's studies showed how authorities laboriously instilled disciplinary norms of health into the social body, what is striking about the neoliberal context is that health is now deemed to be a goal actively and freely embraced by autonomous subjects. Nikolas Rose describes some of the tenets of this discourse as follows:

Consumers are constituted as actors seeking to maximize their "quality of life" by assembling a "life-style" through acts of choice in a world of goods . . . Healthy bodies and hygienic homes may still be a public value and a political objective. But we no longer need state bureaucracies to enjoin healthy habits of eating, of personal hygiene, of tooth care, and the like, with compulsory inspection, subsidised incentives to eat or drink correctly, and so forth. In the new domain of consumption, individuals will *want* to be healthy, experts will instruct them on how to be so, and entrepreneurs will exploit and enhance this market for health. Health will be ensured through a combination of the market, expertise, and a regulated autonomy.[38]

Social and economic relations are governed through the market, in this view, by means of autonomous choices made by self-steering individuals. But the noteworthy point about this context is that the rhetoric of freedom does not quite saturate the social field. In 1984 Milton and Rose Friedman wrote in favor of the decriminalization of drugs on the basis of consumer choice, for example—a move that, as John Clarke points out, "it is difficult to imagine the evangelists or the neo-conservative ideologues going along with."[39]

Eve Sedgwick has expressed something of the conundrum that neo-liberalism represents for queer critique:

Writing in 1988—that is, after two full terms of Reaganism in the United States—D. A. Miller proposes to follow Foucault in demystifying "the intensive and continuous 'pastoral' care that liberal society proposes to take of each and every one of its charges." As if! I'm a lot less worried about being pathologized by my shrink than about my vanishing mental health coverage—and that's given the great good luck of having health insurance at all. Since the beginning of the tax revolt, the government of the United States—and, increasingly, those of other so-called liberal democracies—has been positively rushing to divest itself of answerability for care to its charges (cf. "entitlement programs")—with no other institutions proposing to fill the gap.[40]

These comments seem particularly pertinent in the current Australian context, where state policies have gradually been undermining a comparatively progressive, state-supported, "community response" to AIDS (to name just one social program). In this context, there is a justified hankering for the security of the welfare state. But "even the illiberal liberal state maintains a certain investment in 'pastoral care,'" as Paul Morrison remarks of the Sedgwick passage.[41] One of the alarming features of the right agenda, for example, is the steady rise of a prohibitory morality in drug policy. This has taken place despite the undeniably positive role that harm reduction measures, such as the institution of needle and syringe exchanges, have played in Australia in terms of averting a large-scale HIV epidemic among injecting drug users. According to governmentality scholars, the shrinking state replaces the moral agenda of "discipline" with a more "efficient," "amoral" focus on the correlates of risk.[42] How, then, are we to explain this steady rise in prohibitory morality on the part of a state dead set on shrinking?

This book argues that discourses on the proper use of drugs compose a site at which medical subjectivity and consumer activity are locked together to constitute a misleading vision of moral safety. By this, I do not mean to suggest that the use of drugs is risk-free. Rather, the point is that the regulation of drugs has become a symbolic site at which ideological lessons about the propriety of consumption are propounded. Drugs are curious things. Their use is perfectly intelligible within the neoliberal context as a mode of consumer pleasure, but it is also subject to strict legal sanctions and forceful interdiction. These measures are carried out in the name of safety, but often they have little to do with safety. Frequently they are shown to make practices of drug consumption more unsafe, not less. This contradiction is a paradox that is *lying at the heart* of neoliberal projections of healthy citizenship. In practice, this formulation of healthy citizenship has very little time for the actual bodies impacted by drugs. Where the discourse of compliance dissolves into notions of autonomous selfhood and contractual individuality (so that the shortcomings of medications become a putative effect of "personal choice"), the motif of correct consumption embodied in the discourse of drug abuse remains embedded in law, where it becomes available for the state to deploy it in a spectacular and opportunistic fashion. This gives rise to an exercise of power which can be characterized as "exemplary power" because it is undertaken more as a symbolic demonstration of sovereign authority than for any practical purpose with respect to drug harm.

How to understand the political appropriation of medicine that takes place under the aegis of drugs? Medical subjectivity attains a special significance in the context of the consumer culture of the last quarter of the twentieth century because it configures a *self* as the responsible minister of consuming conduct and medical concern. Discourses on drugs become an important arena through which relations and conduct within consumer culture are imagined as being contained at the level of bodies, subjects, and nations. A medico-moral discourse on drugs is invested with the task of securing the body—as normal, in control, and stable—against the licensed pleasures of the market. But this image of control is under increasing pressure as medicine itself becomes subject to a consumerist logic, so that the distinction between treatment and enhancement becomes blurred, and medicine is wrenched away from the restorative function that is thought to ground its moral authority. The result is an ever-more-insistent performance of concern for drug control, pursued for purposes that are more symbolic than they are "medically" effective. Official discourses of drug use evoke a space within which a violent clash between a moral state and an amoral market is imagined as contained. In the early chapters of this book I track the emergence of this disciplinary investment in drug regimes. In later chapters, I turn to the field of gay men's health promotion and HIV prevention to examine some of the challenges of conducting what might be termed *counterpublic health* in this context.

A BACKDROP TO THIS BOOK is the queer party culture in Sydney in the 1990s, which provided one of the formative contexts of my adult life. This geographic and historical location affords a particular perspective on the relation between health and pleasure that could be of more than local interest. The Australian policy response to AIDS is justly acclaimed for having recognized, relatively quickly, the importance of involving the groups most affected by the epidemic in shaping a viable policy response. From the start, it positioned those minoritized groups as necessary partners in the creation and delivery of educational programs and policy. The approach that emerged rejected many of the coercive medical and state measures that had been promoted within traditional approaches to public health, emphasizing instead community education, participation, and civil rights.[43] The styles of education that developed within this framework set out to address sexual subcultures in their own language and imagery, while adopting a sex-positive approach to education and prevention. In the field of drug policy, government supported harm-reduction measures such as the provision of needle and syringe exchanges, which went against the grain of a prohibitionist stance on drugs. As a result, and in stark contrast to other countries, Australia averted a major HIV epidemic among injecting drug users, while infection rates among gay men (who in Australia comprise the vast majority of HIV infections) dropped substantially and remained low for well over a decade.

The official response to HIV/AIDS took shape at almost precisely the same time that gay, lesbian, and transgender cultures were acquiring newfound public visibility through the annual Mardi Gras celebrations in Sydney. When the first cases of AIDS were reported among gay men in the United States in 1983, Mardi Gras was only just transforming from its origins in 1978 as a violent clash between police and a motley crew of gay liberationists, bar patrons, and other assorted queers who were out on the streets paying tribute to Stonewall.[44] When government officials first met with gay activists to discuss how best to respond to the epidemic, Mardi Gras was on the way to becoming the country's most popular street parade, an annual fixture that would dynamize and generally enliven Australian public and counterpublic culture. In an important sense, the parade became the vehicle through which the possibility of a creative community response to the epidemic was realized, primarily through spectacular and irreverent floats which dramatized the exuberance and scale of such a collective project. Mardi Gras became practically synonymous with this public expression of pleasure and defiance. It signalled the vibrant possibility of life exceeding AIDS—the radical synergies implicit in the political possibility of combining care *and* pleasure.

Mardi Gras grew into a hyperbolic annual street parade complete with arts festival and extravagant dance party—a tourist magnet attracting mainstream sponsors, political endorsement, and international attention.[45] But the closing years of the twentieth century saw a marked loss of interest in the dance party—a form that had come to comprise one of the primary sources of independent revenue for gay and lesbian cultural, political, and health institutions. The subsequent insolvency crisis of the Sydney Gay and Lesbian Mardi Gras in 2002 echoed similar events in other gay urban centers around the world, spelling a significant challenge for gay and lesbian cultural and political initiatives. Mardi Gras had been the source of—and subject to—many transformations over the years. How then to understand this nearly fatal episode in its history?

I want to consider the operation of drugs in the changing nature of the dance-party form, as part of an attempt to offer an alternative framework for conceiving their corporeal and historical effects. Drugs have been a significant part of these gay practices of transformation and self-creation—though it has been unclear how to grasp their activity. The higher rates of substance use among sexual minorities are typically seen as a pathological response to the ingrained violence of homophobia and social alienation. But this perspective does not quite capture the role that drugs play in distinctive practices of sociability, belonging, and pleasure.[46] If one is prepared, on the other hand, to suspend the conventional narrative of victimization and allow drugs a more constituent role in the shaping of culture, it is still not easy to conceive how chemistry might participate in cultural production and transformation. Where pharmacological determinism imputes a fixed and essential set of effects to the biochemical activity of drugs, cultural scholars seek to approach biology as an always already meaningful social force. I want to argue to this effect that drugs are significant social actors with effects which frequently exceed common assignments of value, harm, effect, and productivity. But if drugs do complicate distinctions between the biological and the social, they do so in ways that are rarely predictable and often surprising, as a consideration of the queer dance party illustrates.

The Death of the Dance Party?

The queer dance party is often seen as a sort of mass escape from the realities of queer life or else a scene of excessive consumerism. But I want to suggest that it had a series of effects that were more materially productive. If the dance party formed a major source of revenue for community-based organizations, it was also a crucial apparatus within which the notion of community was given popular resonance—indeed became widely imaginable as a viable way of contending with the HIV/AIDS epidemic. To entertain this idea, we need to consider that "community" is not simply a preexisting entity out of which politics and culture somehow naturally spring, but that it is actively made and apprehended through the historical and embodied forms through which it constitutes and recognizes itself. In *The Motion of Light in Water*, Samuel Delaney writes of his first visit to St Mark's Bathhouse in New York in 1963. The dimly lit sight of an "undulating mass of naked male bodies, spread wall to wall" gives him a new "sense of political power."[47] This is not because of its intimation of a "cornucopia of sexual plenty," but rather because it cast the history of homosexuality in an altogether new light. Though he had participated in similar scenes before in darker and more concealed conditions, on this occasion the dim blue lights, the gym-sized room, the sheer mass of bodies allow him to imagine an altogether different history from that implied by the image of the isolated pervert. "The first direct sense of political power," he writes, "comes from the apprehension of massed bodies."[48]

In an influential essay, "Experience," Joan Scott uses this account to illustrate the now common poststructuralist proposition that the truth of experience does not exist independently of our means of access to it. According to Scott, for Delaney this event

> marked what in one kind of reading we would call a coming to consciousness of himself, a recognition of his authentic identity, one he had always shared, would always share with others like himself. Another kind of reading . . . sees this event not as the discovery of truth (conceived as the reflection of a prediscursive reality), but as the substitution of one interpretation for another. . . . Moreover "the properties of the medium through which the visible appears—here, the dim blue light, whose distorting, refracting qualities produce a wavering of the visible," make any claim to unmediated transparency impossible. Instead, the wavering light permits a vision beyond the visible, a vision that contains the fantastic projections ("millions of gay men" for whom "history had, actively and already, created . . . whole galleries of institutions") that are the basis for political identification.[49]

In Scott's analysis, the vision of the bathhouse is not the transparent revelation of some truth about identity, but an event that makes it possible for Delany to see, understand, imagine differently. Nor is it merely a matter of representation, if representation is understood as arbitrary—

capable of being willed into existence or willed away at whim. As this example makes clear, the experience involves physical structures and technical procedures—the room, the light bulb, the moving bodies, the diary form in which the memory is recorded: the distinct practices and conditions of perception that make up all discourse, knowledge, and imagination.

What if we were to understand the dance party not as the transparent radiation of community, but as a mediated event through which a sense of community was hallucinated? The massed bodies, decorations, lights, drugs, costumes, and music combined to produce a powerful and widely accessed perception of presence, belonging, shared circumstance, and vitality at a time when the image of the gay man, dying alone, ostracized from family, was the publicly proffered alternative. To describe this experience as hallucination is not to say that it was false or untrue, for this would be to imply, incorrectly, that there is some pure, unmediated reality which it is possible to access transparently. I want to take seriously the importance of pleasure, imagination, and fantasy in the construction of new materialities. The sense of community that was animated at dance parties was real with real effects. It was realized in the affirmative apprehension of thousands of bodies presumed affected in similar ways by the accidents of history and the exclusions of heterosexual society.[50] It was worked out in the minutiae of caring practices, the forging of dependable relations outside the family form, the inventive expression of memory and grief, the commitment to a safe-sex ethic. It was tapped into by agencies seeking to advance the public rights of gay men, lesbians, and people with HIV/AIDS, as well as to deliver health programming and to conduct research. It helped sustain a collective sense of predicament, power, care, and commitment—a shared ethos enabling wide-ranging cooperation and transformative activity. Each of these activities depended for its existence on having "community" as an intelligible construct: a source of popular conviction and collective feeling (and against the odds of 1980s individualism). The dance party comprised a popularly accessible assemblage—a concatenation of bodies, discourses, affects, and artifice that made the sensation of community "mighty real," to borrow a phrase from Sylvester, in both its impact and its effects.[51]

Moira Gatens has written that the political imagination is always attached to bodies—distinct, specifically engendered bodies—and this would be no less true of dance-party bodies.[52] A staple and notorious component of dance parties was of course the recreational use of drugs, in particular ecstasy and its derivatives—which produce quite specifically sensitized bodies. Ecstasy, or methylenedioxymethamphetamine, releases large amounts of serotonin (the neurotransmitter said to control mood) into the synapses, increasing serotonin receptor binding and leading to significant changes in the brain's electrical firing. Though culturally and individually variable, its "most predictable feelings are empathy, openness, peace and caring"[53]—feelings of relaxed euphoria, belonging, interpersonal understanding, and emotional warmth. At dance parties people took ecstasy, bonded, hugged one other, and felt community spirit. And this community spirit was carried over into the day-to-day tasks associated with dealing with an epidemic. It contributed to an overarching frame and structure of feeling—an enabling structure within which a whole range of activities gained meaning and coherence.

Of course, while ecstasy was an important actor in the formation of this community, it was not the only or immediate cause of it. Community was conceived in other domains of discourse, practice, and politics, each interweaving with the dance-party phenomenon in direct and indirect ways. I'm not suggesting that people engaging in community-minded activities needed a constant supply of ecstasy to do so—at least not all of them, all the time. But if the dance party provided a key context in which the notion of community was imagined, practiced, and remembered on a popular scale, and the consumption of ecstasy was one of the biochemical and embodied preconditions of the atmosphere and sensation of these events, it would be foolish to ignore the activity of this biochemical agent in the broader network of meaning and practice. Ecstasy was an active component in the effective community response to AIDS.[54]

This argument should not be seen as amounting to a prescription for ecstasy—to "promote community attachment," as health promoters might put it.[55] Though the effects of this drug are widely shared (and occasionally harmful), they are not meaningful or predictable in a straightforward or linear way. Taking ecstasy does not give an individual an enhanced propensity for fighting AIDS—except in the historical context of the institutions and discourses in which its use was embedded. Its use made sense and acquired value within broader conditions of practice and experience, an observation that brings me to my next point. One of the conditions that made the sensations of ecstasy particularly resonant was precisely the context of the AIDS crisis. While the traffic in ecstasy in the 1980s gave rise to a general culture of partying—the rave and so on—in the queer context the dance party took on a particular significance, becoming one of the central sites within which an empowering sense of community and sexual belonging was both performed and embodied. The wide-scale experience and intuition of death—the death of hundreds of gay men a year—was the backdrop against which the experience of coming together en masse—the presence of thousands of vibrant and sexualized bodies—made a powerful, exciting, and profoundly political statement of resilience and possibility. The halls of the Royal Agricultural Showground in Sydney were steeped in amazement and wonder. The chemically facilitated feelings of togetherness, euphoria, caring, and love took on vivid significance. In addition, the temporality of AIDS— the radically reduced life span an HIV diagnosis meant at that time— generated a variously articulated practical philosophy of living for the moment. While this phrase can (and sometimes did) invoke reckless hedonism, a better way of understanding it is in terms of a pursuit of intensified experientiality, in which the pleasures of the self are appreciably bound up in the nature and quality of relations with others—in practices of care, hope, memory, dance, excitement, and disclosure. In the living, this philosophy generated some pretty wild parties. And recognition of it as a practical frame substantially affecting the atmosphere of dance parties makes it possible to comprehend how drugs may have killed the dance party.

Not the recreational, but the medical sort. If anything, the abundance of recreational drugs kept the large-scale dance party going in comparable forms. But the introduction in the late 1990s of effective medical treatments—combination antiretroviral therapy—profoundly altered the temporality of HIV. We can glean some insight into the sort of impact this had on the affective life of the dance party from an account by David Menadue written in 2002. Menadue describes how the introduction of effective treatments has his system "feeling fairly relaxed about the future, enough to start thinking beyond the old one or two year timeframe which AIDS used to suggest for many of us."[56] Depicting himself as an "extraordinarily regular attendee at Mardi Gras"—"they do act as a kind of 'Gay Christmas' for me, chronicling much of my adult life as a gay man and as a person with HIV"—Menadue finds himself "tied up in psychological knots during some quiet moments on the edge of the party dancefloor" at Mardi Gras in 2002.

> I was contemplating Mardi Gras gone by and thinking about issues like how survival with HIV has changed over the years. . . . For the past few years my dancefloor musings have been less about the incredible luck of my survival and the desperate hope that I would live to see another Mardi Gras with my health relatively unscathed—a common thought for much of the early to mid-nineties for me—and more about supposedly normal things. Like: what am I doing sauntering around Mardi Gras dancefloors in my fiftieth year, admiring but being tortured at the same time by the beautiful young bodies parading before me? In other words, I was preoccupied with the same dilemmas about growing older which I imagine most people entering their sixth decade are thinking about as well, regardless of their HIV status.

For Menadue, this shift in temporal horizons changes the party into an experience of a qualitatively different sort, imbued with different and more general concerns, desires, and emotions. Note that this is not merely understood as an effect of growing older. It also reflects an alteration in the conditions through which a sense of time and finitude come into consciousness.

Walter Benjamin's notion of auratic value helps to understand how the time frames of AIDS affected the culture of the dance party. Benjamin uses the concept of aura to describe the singularity and uniqueness of the work of art prior to the age of mechanical reproduction. This singularity arises from the distance and inaccessibility of the work of art in space and time: there is only one of it, it is hard to get to, and access is steeped in ritual and cult value. "Even the most perfect reproduction of a work of art is lacking in one element: its presence in time and space, its unique existence in the place it happens to be."[57] The singular existence of the work of art "in the place it happens to be" gives it a character of authenticity and authority—the character of individual uniqueness that Benjamin terms *aura*. But in the era of mechanical reproduction, we must reach for other attributes and aspects of a product in order to deliver the same effect.

Now, it may seem that one dance party is very like another. But Menadue's description makes it possible to see how the pre-antiretroviral experience of HIV may have produced each dance party as one of a kind. It contributed to the sense of singularity that I want to call the auratic value of queer dance parties. The mood of a party depends of course on the multi-various activities of the entire mass of its differentiated consumer-producers:[58] the AIDS crisis, in this respect, was only the most intractable of its many historical backdrops. An early-epidemic HIV diagnosis could readily have generated two interrelating optics that take on special significance in such a context: the heightened value attached to repetition and yearly remembrance (the sense of chronicling a life), and the poignant awareness that this party could be the last one. These two temporal frames may have combined to produce the cult value of the queer dance party: the exhilarating sense of singularity and uniqueness that was felt to imbue this experience. One needn't have been actually infected with the virus to have had a palpable appreciation of these meanings, even if only subliminally, given the intense inter-affective mood they inspired. Nor had all partygoers to be adjusting to the new futures enabled by combination antiretroviral therapy for them to have experienced the deflation in atmosphere and ambience that the long-awaited introduction of these pharmaceuticals may have occasioned. If the temporal orientation that characterized the early AIDS crisis delivered the queer dance party up as an experience of an exceptional sort, then in the presence of treatments and their altered temporalities, and under such changed historical conditions, the dance party may well have come to be experienced in terms of lack: as a pale imitation of former years.

There is a further sense in which the recent popular disappointment with queer dance parties convinces me of the aptness of Benjamin's account. Community pundits characterized the changed atmosphere of dance parties in various ways, often perceiving it as a question of scale. Writing evocatively in the *Sydney Star Observer*, for example, Geoff Honnor observed: "There was a time when 3,000 people at a party represented an incredibly powerful statement about being here. And that 20,000 people can be more about the quantity of numbers than it is about the quality of power."[59] And Fiona McGregor's *Chemical Palace*, a finely observed account of the gradual changes that occurred in Sydney's party culture and urban landscape over the 1990s, contains the following passage: "The parties got bigger the tickets more expensive, strangers outnumbered friends the community grew. Splintered multiplied mutated atrophied, sprang up elsewhere. The random march of queer seeding the world. People were always looking for something new, so much good partying led to high standards. There were never enough places to go for aficionados. Rebel parties became institutions."[60] McGregor's prose forces disparate elements into close proximity: they hang together like a Sydney street or else a queer event. On the one hand, changes in scale are experienced as a problem: strangers outnumber friends. But strangers are also enfolded into community here, in a volatile process of growth and mutation. When a visceral sense of belonging has been encountered with complete strangers in a space like the dance party, the torsion between friends and strangers under the sign of community becomes an ambiguous but tangible process. The concept of community is made to strain against the force of given understandings, those that would prescribe a zone of mutual recognition, sameness, and natural intimacy.[61] Of course, strangers have always been a vital part of the excitement and appeal of the big dance parties, bringing us out of our homes to flirt, to dance, to party. What McGregor is conveying here is a subtle recontextualization in the apprehension of the stranger. I am suggesting that what these accounts are registering is not merely an effect of scale, but also a much more subtle and elusive shift. They index a loss of singularity, a transformation from the qualitative to the quantitative, a conversion of auratic value into commodity value.

Benjamin's essay is, in part, a meditation on the commodity form. In his account, the aura of the work of art is challenged, almost fatally, by the advent of technologies that enable the mechanical reproduction of cultural objects. Benjamin hoped that the awe reserved for the unique work of art would decline in this context, so that the democratic possibilities of mass reproduction might be realized. Quite a touching and momentous idea in his essay, however, is that auratic value doesn't just disappear in these conditions, but finds a temporary lodgement in other domains. In the case of film, the aura reconfigures in the cult of the celebrity. In the case of photography, cult value "retires into an ultimate retrenchment: the human countenance . . . the aura emanates from the early photographs in the fleeting expression of a human face. This is what constitutes their melancholy, incomparable beauty."[62] More topically, Sarah Thornton has suggested that the mass reproduction of music embodied in the record relocates the attribution of "authenticity" from the stage to the dance floor, where the aura can be thought to manifest in "the buzz or energy which results from the interaction of record, DJ and crowd"—giving rise to the cult of the DJ.[63] In sum, under conditions of mechanical reproduction we come to invest new aspects of the cultural product with the task of delivering upon the culturally rampant desire for authenticity and immediacy.

Now, dance parties are a commodity par excellence, and ever were— an interactive scene involving multiple (some would say excessive) forms of cultural consumption, repeated in time and space, with a predictable formula and very expensive tickets. I have argued here however that the distinctive temporality of the crisis produced the queer dance party as an experience that seemed especially significant, even in repetition. The curtailed futures of AIDS seemed to lift the dance party out of the circumstances of its mass reproduction, providing a broad frame (not the only one, by any means) through which its uniqueness was constituted. With the transformation in these conditions, then, it's not surprising that the dance party comes to lose something of its aura. The party gets stripped bare, reduced to the thinly veiled machinery of mechanical reproduction. Its yearly repetition no longer bears a special poignancy, but smacks of seriality. The undulating mass no longer appears as a diverse community bound together by a singular sensibility, but takes the shape of a chaotic and alienating crowd. The congregation of bodies is no longer "an incredibly powerful statement about being here," but an aggregate of individual consumers. The dance party starts to manifest "the phony spell of a commodity."[64]

The insolvency of Mardi Gras formed the occasion for an intense round of public debate, a recurrent theme of which was that Mardi Gras had become "too commercial." In this view, Mardi Gras had lost touch with its roots, and—whether through commercialization, mismanagement, or sheer size—had become an impersonal and alienating experience. The dance party took the shape of a particularly loathsome *bête noire* in this discourse. Apart from embodying the politically unpalatable image of gay men as consummate consumers, unvirtuously frittering their incomes away on party drugs and gym memberships, it seemed somehow to encapsulate people's sense of alienation and exclusion from their community institutions: the perceived loss of political resonance. A hankering for "community" and "transparency" was the thematic resolution to these overtures—a move that saw "community" set up in contradistinction to "commerce" and operating as a siphon for people's frustrated desires to access some purified experience of communal presence and belonging. New Mardi Gras, an alliance of community-based organizations, successfully channelled these desires into support for its vision of a leaner, more inclusive, more "community" version of Mardi Gras, stripped of all overt and explicit trappings of the market.

But New Mardi Gras cannot plausibly claim to be the utopian alternative to commerce. It anticipates a turnover of several million dollars. A political appraisal of this moment cannot, at any rate, simply content itself with the charge of commodification. If the large-scale queer dance party is a form in decline, this is not simply because it became more commercial, but because one of the primary conditions within which it came to accrue meaning and value has altered—and thankfully so. The discourse and sensation of community, which was initially and ecstatically embodied at these events against the terrible backdrop of the AIDS crisis, has come back in an intense but barely recognized form: as a displaced but powerful *memory* of community, haunting and obfuscating the Mardi Gras postmortem. The complaints of commercialization and alienation that pervaded this discourse are the trace of the intense relationality whose fabrication was once necessary to survive the crisis—a relationality now understandably mourned.[65] Realizing the power of this memory calls, not for nostalgia, but for the formation of further counterpublic spaces and connections.[66]

Indeed, there's a question of whether "community" is even the best way to conceive collective political efforts around queer health and well-being today. As Judith Halberstam has discussed, there is a nostalgia built into the very concept that may prevent recognition of the queer possibilities that inhere in the present.[67] The concept is increasingly used by the mainstream gay and lesbian movement to promote a normalizing agenda. With its intonations of a prior moment of pure belonging, the concept of community hankers after a wholesome past, all the while trying to forget its strange and checkered history (at least, if the history of the dance party is any indication!). All too often, "community" is used to separate out the moral sheep from the goats, in tactics that are frequently disingenuous, exclusionary, self-sanitizing, and damaging. The recent construction of crystal methamphetamine use among gay men is a particularly fraught example. To my mind, any concept of collective activity that is fit for addressing the complex challenges of queer health, pleasure, and well-being in any inclusive sense today needs to question those routine acts of purification that separate out the biological from the social, the licit from the illicit, the natural from the artificial, the organic from the technical, the wholesome from the depraved, and ethics from embodiment in its imagination of present possibility.[68]

This reading of the dance party raises questions for concrete inquiry, questions about how the relations of the market inflect cultural and political possibilities, and about the constitution of political, cultural, and remembering bodies. But these questions will not be usefully answered by partitioning off some bodies as pristine. Indeed, Benjamin might be read to suggest that the forceful dismemberment and reconfiguration of auratic value has a broader political applicability. An arbitrary and potentially violent swing between the designation of the authentic or natural, and the designation of the inauthentic or artificial, may be a perennial feature of existence in commodity culture—and ever available for political deployment. What the discourse surrounding the insolvency of Mardi Gras illustrates is how quickly and deceptively drugs and their metonyms can turn into fetishized symbols of all that is experienced as artificial, inauthentic, alienating, and untrue—always capable of implying a purer, unmediated, natural space that claims to exist before consumption, politics, and contest. But this space conceived as natural does not innocently exist, which raises the pressing question of who or what gets crushed or distorted in the mad rush to occupy the space of the natural? As Helen Keane has argued, even "in the realm of neuroscience, the distinction between the natural and the chemical breaks down, because the brain is itself chemical."[69] Neither community nor brain are completely self-enclosed systems—whether on or off drugs. What drugs therefore also supply is a useful model for thinking about how our perception of the real, the authentic, the healthy, the true, is impossible to extricate from the dense, interpenetrating, embodied circumstances—

those historical, cultural, and biochemical conditions of mediation—through whose means we gain even the most sober access to it.[70]

Drugs can be approached as an attempt, on the part of users, to construct new materialities in the context of specific embodied circumstances and normative regimes. But they are also subject to new modes of power within the current biosocial order. Against these disciplinary interventions, I suggest that the transformations, pleasures, and forms of enablement, disablement, and escape found in drugs should be approached more simply as experimental and material engagements with the circumstances of life.

2

PRESCRIBING THE SELF

. . .

In acclimatizing to the discourses and demands of new treatment regimens, gay men with HIV experienced a significant shift in their experience of temporality. The discourse of compliance can be seen to reorient temporality and embodiment to elicit a prudent subject, more concerned with "supposedly normal things," like aging, responsibility, and normativity.[1] One of the aims of this book is to take stock of this reorientation, which, among other things, expresses a changing relation between gay men, illness, and the medical establishment. When I started this project, two discourses concerning drug use were radically reconfiguring the scope of responses to HIV: a discourse of patient compliance, which concerned the use of antiretroviral medication to treat HIV illness, and a discourse of drug abuse, which, apart from providing a basis for moral censure in its own right, was more and more frequently offered as an explanation for sexual risk-taking and thus for the continuation of the epidemic among gay men. One of the effects of these discourses was to transfer official proposals of how to respond to the epidemic away from any notion of collective interactivity and commitment and to locate them squarely in the therapeutic context. The way forward, from this perspective, was a matter of individual moral compliance, rather than the sort of collective elaboration and sexual creativity that had informed the development of safe sex and that had proven highly effective—indeed groundbreaking—as a public health response. The creativity of the initial gay response to HIV/AIDS (which did not condemn the use of illicit drugs as a matter of policy) suggests that compliant subjectivity is not the only version of responsibility capable of addressing the experience of risk, nor necessarily the most effective. In order to better understand how discourses of drug use reorient subjectivity and circumscribe agency, however, it is worth undertaking some historical work and asking some questions, such as how do drug discourses connect subjectivity to broader normative structures? How does the discourse of compliance set out to discipline the encounters of bodies, authorities, and drugs—and with what effects?

To address these questions, a more general genealogy of patient compliance is needed, as well as an investigation of the corresponding discourse of drug abuse, with a view to considering the significance these discourses acquire in the context of the broader political and economic shifts associated with neoliberalism. Obviously, medical, political, and public health regimes vary considerably from state to state. What is interesting here are certain broad transformations in Western expert discourses on drugs over the twentieth century, so my archive draws liberally from North American, UK, and Australian medical and legal discussions, while attempting to highlight some of the different conceptions that have emerged.[2] This approach emphasizes the shifting "problematizations" of drugs and drug conduct: I try to open the "drug problem" out into its multiplicity and various socio-historical coordinates. The study of problematizations directs attention to the historical terms "through which being offers itself to be, necessarily, thought—and the practices on the basis of which these problematizations are formed."[3] It traces the systems of judgment, images, and ideals according to which certain situations become "matters of concern," in an attempt to dismantle commonsense understandings and indicate the multiplicity of possible responses within given sets of constraints.

The Subject of Compliance

Compliance with Therapeutic Regimens, published in 1976, is one of the earliest reference texts on the topic of compliance. David Sackett, a professor of clinical epidemiology, introduces the volume as follows:

> The gap between the therapy prescribed by the clinician and the therapy actually taken by the patient is distressingly wide for self-administered regimens. However, it is one of the paradoxes of non-compliance that the therapist is frequently the last to know. . . . For many students of compliance, an initial awareness of the extent of noncompliance came in the form of awestruck disbelief at reading the

work of pioneers such as [A. B.] Bergman and [R. J.] Werner in North America and [Alan] Porter in Great Britain. As more reports have appeared it has become apparent that noncompliance is a protean feature of all therapeutic regimens that involve self-administration.[4]

Compliance is defined in this text as "the extent to which the patient's behavior (in terms of taking medications, following diets, or executing other life-style changes) coincides with the clinical prescription."[5] Sackett frames noncompliance as an issue of natural concern for the clinician, positing the phenomenon as a recent discovery at the hands of intrepid pioneers. More reports, we are told, have come in, confirming the worst fears of those at the frontline, the concerned folk back home, and the students of the discipline so constituted, "that noncompliance is a protean feature of all therapeutic regimens that involve self-administration." Following doctors' advice is localized as a discrete behavior—one that is measurable, explainable, and transformable by the work of a team of experts: researchers, educators, counselors, and others.

The illustration that accompanies the announcement for the symposium on which *Compliance with Therapeutic Regimens* is based—placed, we are told, in "the appropriate journals"—depicts an explosive scene: a busy landscape filled with unruly pill-popping characters (see figure 1). One woman, smiling soporifically, reaches for a container of pills and wonders, "How about a pretty blue and white one?" A mother clasps her child in a headlock, forcing medication into the girl's tightly clenched jaw. Other characters grimace, shrug, or smirk as they throw pills down their throats. One boy grins mischievously as he smuggles pills into the mouth of his appreciative dog. There is even a man in a YMCA tank top, who makes a disheartened expression as he stands on a scale. In the top left-hand corner a scientist stands perched atop a pile of boxes marked "Ajax Pillco." With a menacing smile, he lights a huge cannon, jettisoning bodies across the top right-hand corner in a magnificent explosion of pharmaceutical products. Some mouths are forced open, while others gape to catch the drugs propelled their way. The disarray is so great that one of the British journals refused to run the advertisement, the authors report.[6] Even in the representing, this mayhem is staged as far too much for the more staid corridors of medicine.

These constitutive acts are important; they give insight into the terms

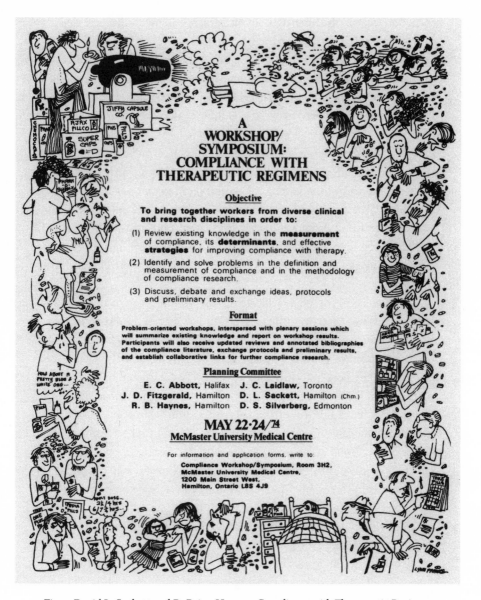

Fig. 1. David L. Sackett and R. Brian Haynes, *Compliance with Therapeutic Regimens* (Baltimore: Johns Hopkins University Press, 1976), Figure 1, "A Workshop/Symposium: Compliance with Therapeutic Regimens." © 1976 Johns Hopkins University Press. Reprinted with permission of the Johns Hopkins University Press.

according to which this new body of research is made to seem signifi-cant. The sense of clinicians aghast at this unforeseen discovery, the assignation of "pioneers" and "students," the conviction that diverse practices are explicable under the one rubric—these things help legiti-mate a new object of research. Perhaps more intriguing, though, is the role clinicians are invited to occupy. Following doctors' orders is cast as a distinct species of normal behavior from which it is possible to deviate. And delinquency is precisely the register of concern. The gap between what we assumed and what actually goes on is "*distressingly* wide." "An initial awareness of the extent" of the problem is met with "awestruck disbelief." "The therapist is frequently the last to know." At a time when society is recoiling from the explosive cultural upheavals of the sixties, clinicians are invited to occupy the subjectivity of naïve but concerned parents, shocked to their senses by grim reports of their charges' un-seemly behavior.

The imagery of compliance bespeaks a nervous relation to an energetic field of consumer activity—the women's movement, self-help, consumer-health activism, and countercultural body politics. Through a discourse on the proper use of drugs, compliance brings this activity within the purview of medical authority and concern. Two explanations are com-monly given for the burgeoning interest in patient compliance. The first associates it with the use of the survey in clinical practice, placing its inception alongside the appearance of the "defaulting patient" in the 1930s.[7] The second attributes it to the wide availability, in the 1950s, of effective medications.[8] But it is not until the 1970s that compliance research really takes off. And explosion is certainly the best way to describe the production of its literature at this time. A cumulative bibli-ography on the subject lists 22 articles published in English before 1960, and 850 published by 1978.[9] A search on Medline reveals 6 articles published between 1960 and 1969, 1,519 between 1970 and 1979, an astounding 6,480 articles in the 1980s, and 9,096 in the 1990s. Though they form important preconditions, the given explanations do not suffi-ciently account for the growth of interest in patient compliance, nor the terms in which it is offered to thought. Rather, the remarkable upsurge in compliance literature bears a crucial relation to a broader way of under-standing and grounding social conduct that takes shape at this time. It signals a new operationalization of medical authority and a new object of medical concern. To understand how and why this is so, it is necessary to pay particular attention to the formulation of the new behavior: "non-compliance is a protean feature of all therapeutic regimens that involve self-administration." The phrase is as broad in designation as it is ambiguous. We are not sure whether noncompliance is a problem of patient conduct or a property of drug regimens. It could very well be both. There is a curious slippage, a strong ambiguity, in whether it is something new in the nature of the therapies available, or something new about patient behavior, that best explains the new research interest. The cartoon places the ballooning rate of commercial production in the picture, but the behavior in question is conspicuous for the way it exceeds the simple consumption of pharmaceutical commodities. Compliance is imagined to pertain to a whole range of activities—from following diets to wearing seatbelts, from brushing teeth to attending rehabilitation programs and exercising (remember our YMCA friend from the cartoon?). All these things are said to be the same, suddenly interesting, phenomenon. Taking medicine comprises only a portion of the topic. Indeed, drugs seem to be performing the role of a protean and cautionary signifier for all sorts of "life-style changes."

Perhaps the new drugs act as a projected surface onto which the problem of "self-administration" is articulated. For it is self-administration that provides the frame through which these diverse activities are offered to thought as a *problem requiring attention*. The increased availability of pharmaceutical products makes it possible to think of these practices in terms of their alignment with medical advice. "Self-administration" makes the various activities cohere. At the same time, self-administration becomes subject to a particular sort of scrutiny, with medicine acting as a distinct point of reference. In what follows, I approach the remarkable upsurge in compliance literature as evidence of a new problematization of self-activity in which drugs play a significant role. My point is not simply that compliance operates as an ideology that shores up doctors' authority—a familiar enough argument in the anti-medicine literature.[10] Indeed, the doctor all but disappears in the emerging articulation of research science, the patient-consumer, and pharmaceutical production that begins to take shape from the 1980s on. Rather, this chapter begins to trace the emergence of a new field of normativity around health and consumption, in which the moral worth of subjects is *exemplified* in relation to a generalized sense of medical prescription.

Prescription

With respect to pharmacologically active substances, then, it appears that self-administration is a relatively recent invention. Here I am not referring to a point in history at which people started to consume such substances by themselves, but rather to the period in which "self-administration" appears as an object of concern in medical practice, articulated through questions of drug use. In order to disentangle what makes up the present sense of "self-administration," it is first necessary to examine how prescription came to acquire the particular authority it possesses—how it came to configure particular relations between doctors, patients, and drugs.

Personal medication, independent of prescription, was a common practice in the nineteenth century. A wide range of therapeutic substances was readily available from doctors, chemists, and even grocers and corner shops. These came in the form of formulary drugs (which were preparations whose composition and technique of manufacture were listed in pharmaceutical compendiums) and "proprietary" or "patent" drugs (which were made from secret ingredients and sold by companies under trademarked names like Irish Moss or Lydia Pinkham's Vegetable Compound). Ingredients commonly included opiates, alcohol, ether, and a range of substances of more dubious therapeutic value. Thus, though doctors have been giving advice and constructing health regimens for centuries, a prescription was only one way (and a relatively unusual one at that) to obtain a drug for treatment until well into the twentieth century. As many historians point out, use of drugs in the nineteenth century was a matter of personal preference, a decision that sometimes (though rarely) relied upon the advice of a doctor.[11]

If consumption, including the consumption of drugs, was a matter of "individual choice" at this time, it was not, however, the "individual choice" of the present moment in the history of consumption. These were not choices made by consumers "seeking to maximize their 'quality of life' by assembling a 'life-style' through acts of choice in a world of

goods," as Nikolas Rose characterizes contemporary practices of the consuming self.[12] Most commonly, drugs were purchased at this time as a
remedy to a variety of common ailments. They were sought as a way of
dealing with sleeplessness or relieving pain, or for just getting by. To be
sure, "luxuriant" or "stimulant" use of opiates in literary and middle-
class society existed, but as Virginia Berridge and Griffin Edwards discuss, personal medication was the most common reason for opiate use,
and though working-class use could well have what we now call "recreational" effects, drugs were not usually taken with such effects in mind.[13]

If doctors' advice was rarely accessed and had none of the binding
character with which it is imbued today, how did the prescription come
to occupy the authoritative status it now enjoys? Two events laid the
tracks for the present sense of medical prescription. First, expertise—
including medical expertise—came to be articulated into the apparatus
of liberal rule in a particular way, one that depended upon the mechanism of the state license. Second, the category of "prescription drugs"
was enshrined in legislature. These events were unrelated and, when they
occurred, served purposes that were quite different to how they later
came to function.[14] Yet their coexistence allowed the formation of a particular institution, that of prescription, that takes on major importance
for the authority of doctors over the course of the twentieth century.

Industrialization in the nineteenth century created a variety of disturbances that accorded expertise a new form of authority. Independent
reformers, experts, and professionals enlisted political, legal, and organi-
zational resources to deal with some of the consequences of industrialization: epidemics, pauperism, and other effects of the new environment
of human relations. These problems came to be encoded as "social." In
the process a particular relation between expertise and liberal government began to develop in which both were bound together. State licensing was sought and granted to various professional bodies, among them
doctors and pharmacists. Licensing acted as a way of securing members'
economic, occupational, and social position in communities that were
changing rapidly. It granted protection to professions at a time when
changes in communication and transport were radically altering the
situation of trade, from the local to the national domain. In so doing,
it accorded experts a particular place in the governmental apparatus.
Through them, the state could secure and "instrumentalize expert capac-

ities (and vice versa) without compromising their independence, truth values, or the autonomy of the domains over which their authority was to run."[15] As Nikolas Rose points out, this is less a case of state intervention, or government extending its tentacles throughout society, than a piecemeal set of independent initiatives that coalesce around particular problems and contribute to a situation in which everyday life comes to be governed through "society."

Even with the existence of licensed practitioners, personal medication was an extremely common practice. Medical prescription did not operate as an exclusive means of obtaining drugs, nor of classifying them. There is evidence that pharmacists copied formulae from the doctors' prescriptions that came into their hands, thus transforming ingredients into a sought-after remedy that was sold to other customers, circumventing trade from the medical profession. Since many doctors dispensed their own drugs, they had their own tricks, such as repackaging patent medicines in plain bottles and writing the name in Latin to retain the trade of customers who might otherwise buy the medicines without their aid.[16] In any event, prescription had little of the exclusive moral force it later came to assume. The relative impotency of prescription is attested in early North American food and drug legislation, the thrust of which was to eliminate the adulteration and misbranding of food and drugs. Nothing in these acts limited the availability of particular drugs by requiring a prescription.[17] The intention, rather, was to maintain the integrity of the food supply in conditions where the increasing competition brought about by the gradual shift from local to national market institutions encouraged practices of food manufacturing as unsavory as they were fraudulent. In relation to drugs, this strategy attempted to combat the secrecy of the ingredients and the dishonesty of advertising practices, rather than attempting to restrict certain drugs. Proper labeling and the accuracy of what manufacturers said about their products were the goals of legislators' efforts. The presupposition here was that the decision to use a particular drug rested with the consumer, who was therefore to be furnished with accurate information.

As food and drug labeling provisions became more onerous and drugs more difficult to describe, manufacturers sought to exclude some of the products entirely from the jurisdiction of regulatory legislation—specifically those they delivered solely to doctors. In the U.S. Food, Drug, and Cosmetic Act of 1938, some exemptions from the labeling require-ments were allowed for drugs that were prescribed by licensed medical practitioners. Drugs labeled "Caution: To be used only by or on the prescription of a physician" and delivered only to physicians were to be free from the information demands of the Act. As part of these provi-sions, a specific requirement that prescription drugs were to be labeled "in such medical terms as are not likely to be understood by the ordinary individual" was enshrined in law. As Peter Temin writes, the prescrip-tion provisions "allow[ed] the drug companies to create a class of drugs that cannot legally be sold without a prescription by putting the appro-priate label on them. This [was] a stunning change in the way drugs were to be sold."[18] For the first time, consumers were obliged to consult a doctor to obtain non-narcotic drugs. Remarkably, the impetus came not from government regulators, as one might expect, but from industry seeking to circumvent demanding labeling requirements. Drug classi-fication, along with the determination of which drugs were to be ob-tained by prescription, was a decision made at the discretion of the drug companies, rather than any "universal" assessment of particular drugs or the risks entailed in their use.

Unwittingly, the new restrictions created a highly prized commodity. Drug companies quickly discovered that "the best way to promote a drug is to advertise that it is used by physicians."[19] Mysteriously, drugs with the deliberately uninformative prescription labeling continued to find their way directly to consumers through nonprescription sales. Though captivated by the glow of a doctor's recommendation, it seemed con-sumers were quite willing to bypass the actual visit to the doctor to obtain medications—and proprietors quite happy to oblige them. Thus, though originally intended to improve and facilitate safe personal medi-cation, the provisions ended up undermining it. Upon the realization that consumers were being deprived, more than ever, of label informa-tion thought to be essential to safe and efficacious use, authorities re-sponded with tighter controls, including assuming the function of desig-nating which drugs fell into the prescription-only category. According to Temin, rather than being grounded in a policy of linking certain drugs exclusively to doctors' authority, the determination of which drugs were to be limited to prescription was originally taken over by government in order to clean up the mess caused by the original restrictions.

As arbitrary, clumsy, or scandalous as this sequence of events appears, it seems it was justified at the time in terms of a broader discourse of maximizing the availability of drugs while safeguarding the consumer—the assumption being that some potent drugs were of great value but dangerous in the hands of those unskilled in their use.[20] Early food and drug legislators were attempting to respond to a problem that continues to be important: how best to inform citizens about the effects and uses of potentially dangerous new technologies, namely pharmaceutical compounds. The solutions proposed had far-reaching implications, not simply for how this was to be done, but also in terms of binding the use of drugs to medical authority. A class of drugs was linked exclusively to the doctor's consultation, and labeled in "such medical terms as are not likely to be understood by the ordinary individual."[21] This allowed particular information channels to coagulate at the node of the doctor's office.[22] Doctors, rather than consumers, became the repository of information on how to use the wonder drugs of later decades. Indeed, consumers were specifically denied intelligible label information on the safe and proper use of drugs. The fortification of prescription in prewar regulation (and well before the antibiotic revolution of the 1940s and 1950s) also had a marked effect on the authority accorded medicine. In their new capacity as access point, doctors accrued the symbolic capital that was afforded by the curative power of these later, more effective medications. Their expertise was vouchsafed by license of government, where previously it had borne no relation, and this license gained new significance as a key to participating in the circulation of drugs. The "authoritative" sense of prescription that emerged—the sense of an expert doctor dispensing knowledge and treatment to the passive and obedient patient—was well fertilized within the rationalities of trust and the formalized relations that were developing between experts and political rule in the context of the welfare state. But the origins of prescription as a category reveal that, in the consumer imagination at least, it was doctors as much as drugs that were authorized in the wake of powerful new treatments. Where previously doctors' advice had been a rare indulgence, admittedly highly valued, but with none of the canonical status it later enjoyed, licensed practitioners now became an essential element in the treatment of illness: a means to remedies (and information about these) that one could not otherwise access. Once an esteemed but rarely elected option, a selection that was valued but hardly binding, the prescription now embodied a powerful and exclusive curative character that one disregarded at one's peril. It took on the character of a mandatory instruction, a staple component of caring for one's health. In short, prescription became a commanding arbiter of social access to health, and doctors a compelling source of authority in the use of drugs.

The Active Patient

At about the same time as this sense of prescription solidifies, its human counterpart emerges. The defaulting patient, the patient who takes medicine the wrong way, is discovered. From the perspective of the clinical and human sciences, this is the form in which the active patient first appears, quite suddenly, in the early twentieth century. Before this time, beyond the patient being a carrier of pathology, his or her subjectivity is all but irrelevant to the clinical gaze. Rarely does the patient's behavior take the form of a topic worth studying or reporting in clinical journals. Thus, though Sackett mentions a recent inception in 1975, the elementary conditions that give rise to the study of "compliance" take shape in the interwar years. In David Armstrong's account of British medicine, it is the discipline of the survey that creates a mechanism for constituting bodies in a fashion quite different from that of the clinic and the hospital. In 1932, the "problem of the defaulter"—a problem investigated by means of questionnaires sent out to patients—accords the patient an initial "germ of idiosyncrasy."[23] Previously a passive body—a corpus of symptoms to be interpreted by the physician—the patient now achieves an identity by virtue of being a potential (and problematic) defaulter. This germ of idiosyncrasy goes on to bloom over the course of the twentieth century into an identity. As the need arises to treat "the patient as other than a wholly passive body, albeit one which, with the correct instructions, could be made passive," the active patient is invented.[24]

Interestingly, some of the earliest research on the question of patient default appears in the *British Journal of Venereal Diseases*. These early studies are intriguing for their decision to single out "the defaulting seaman," "the defaulting prostitute," "the defaulting travelling man," and "the defaulting child" for analysis.[25] The threat perceived in these wayward and itinerant types prompts an extension of the clinical gaze *beyond* the patient as a simple bearer of pathology to include his or her self-medicating activity. Similarly in North America, the quarantine measures at the beginning of the century aimed at containing the threat of tuberculosis transmission give way, with the introduction of antibiotic treatment in the 1940s, to a discourse of patient "recalcitrance." As Barron Lerner explains, patients who "took their outpatient antibiotics inappropriately threatened to squander the outstanding opportunity that the new drugs provided."[26] In the presence of treatments a problem previously associated with certain social classes—"the vagrant, the poor and the immigrant"—transforms into one that emphasizes "the act of disobedience [from doctor's authority] itself."[27] Though still associated with "transient" individuals (usually male alcoholics), the rollout of drugs reconstitutes the problem such that compliance with the medically circumscribed purposes of drugs forms a new and *seemingly* indiscriminate site for embodying responsible personhood.

Default adds new tasks to the doctor's repertoire, such as impressing upon the patient at regular intervals the necessity of treatment, and having patients "repeat all directions so no misunderstanding can occur."[28] Queer and caricatured as the early case studies seem, the emphasis on recalcitrant types continues as the terminology of compliance gains favor. Armstrong refers to compliance as "a much more complex and subtle" discourse than that of default. Initially, compliance levies a greater scrutiny, both on doctor-patient communication, and on the patient's personality. Reflecting a growing interest in medical psychology and the neuroses, the study of compliance is made possible by the enrollment of the psychological and social sciences in the task of investigating non-medical subjectivity. Henry Brackenbury, the secretary of the British Medical Association and author of *Patient and Doctor*, published in 1935, anticipated this trend, stating "the relationship between patient and doctor is not merely, between two persons, but between two personalities," and advocating the location of illness within its social context.[29] No longer just the outcome of sloppy instruction-giving, compliance transforms patient default into a propensity of the "whole person," who is granted complex reasons for not following the therapeutic regimen. The patient gets a personality.

Many differences exist between competing explanations of noncompliance in this literature. A whole branch of this research takes as its focus the patient's personality and attempts to identify the typical traits of non-compliers. It reveals in disappointed tones that authoritative, dependent-submissive, and obstructive patients were as likely as not to misbehave.[30] Reluctant to give up the pursuit of some means of "permitting the elimination of 'irregular patients,'" some researchers attempt to refine techniques to measure the intake of prescribed medications.[31] One study evaluates a Multiphasic Personality Inventory "lie" scale, by means of a bottle count and a tracer technique, in which patients' antacid is laced with bromide.[32] Concerned that patients might catch on, the scientists instruct the delivery man responsible for collecting the empty medicine bottles to "dress like a truck driver and to avoid commenting on the patient's consumption of medication."[33] These "painstaking controls" identify noncompliers among those who obtain normal scores on the personality scale, and the use of personality as a predictor is struck another blow.

Irresistible though these accounts of scientists who dress up or "drag up" to refine their measures may be, studies of this type comprise only a portion of the compliance literature. Perhaps the disciplinary aim of "eliminating irregular patients" provided the necessary backdrop against which practitioners of "softer" approaches could cast their work. Social psychological researchers begin to insist at this time on an examination of the patient in his or her social context. Some point to demographic and attitudinal variables or construe the patient as a rational complex of beliefs, attitudes, and knowledge. Other researchers examine cognitive skills, or locate the problem in doctor-patient communication and inter-action, or advocate tackling the "deep" problem using psychodynamic therapy. The prominent "Health Belief Model" of 1975 tries to explain compliance as the result of complex variations in a unwieldy concoction of beliefs and attributes, comprising motivation, perceived susceptibility to illness, perceived benefits of taking action, psychological barriers, and levels of knowledge of the condition and the therapy. "The 'patient,'" we are informed by its proponents, "is an active participant in dealing with his illness and will take what he regards as appropriate steps within his own life framework."[34]

Meanwhile sociologists and anthropologists adopt social and cultural approaches. Gerry Stimson, a medical sociologist writing in 1973, interprets the study of patient compliance on the part of the harder clinical sciences as "amounting to a moral prescription for patient behaviour" that leads to an "unproductive formulation of the problem of drug use."[35] He proposes "an alternative approach from the perspective of the patient. . . . The focus is then on the social context in which illnesses are lived and treatments used. A more active view of the patient is entailed in which patients have expectations of the doctor, evaluate the doctor's actions, and are able to make their own treatment decisions." His work presages a trend in compliance research that adopts the hermeneutic task of analyzing "the meanings of medication in people's everyday lives."[36] In an article entitled "The Meaning of Medications: Another Look at Compliance," which takes distance from the stauncher psychological explanations such as the health belief model, the sociologist Peter Conrad rejects previous "doctor-centred perspectives," and proclaims that "from a patient's perspective the issue is more one of self-regulation than compliance."[37]

These studies would seem to perform the liberating gesture of studying "the patient as an actor in, rather than a passive recipient of, his own treatment."[38] There is much of value in these studies, which direct attention to the social context of the treatment experience. However, the ubiquity of the assertion that a focus on the active patient will finally redress all that is restrictive about compliance research generates a funny aftertaste. How significant a break is this more "active" view of the patient? What is to be made of the appearance of the active patient to the scientific gaze? Does it mark the (long overdue) recognition on the part of these disciplines that the patient possesses autonomy, is capable of exercising a decision-making power over his or her actions—that the patient is, in short, a subject? Does it represent a challenge to, and potential reform of, paternalistic formulations of the clinical relation? Or is it evidence of an increasing regulation, a surveillance, a desire to discipline this behavior? Is the liberal flourish that greets the great "renaissance" in general practice of the 1960s and 1970s—the rise of "person-centered" medicine—warranted?

If one understands knowledge as arising not in relation to normal conduct but rather in response to conduct and thought deemed troublesome, then the growing number of studies that devote themselves to this question reveals an increasing concern, an intensification of interest, an anxiety about whether the patient will follow medical prescriptions. For all the diversity of explanations of noncompliance and all the inconclusiveness of their findings, these researches share a common feature. It becomes rare to find an article on compliance, regardless of the disciplinary background, that does not insist (as though for the first time) that the patient is active. This insistence appears as a constitutive feature of the object of study. Indeed, every insistence on patient agency on the part of humanist critique ends up being captured by the initial discourse that takes this agency as its theme and problem. Thus, much of the research is undertaken with the intention of helping patients follow their prescriptions. Compliance is a topic that claims to reform itself endlessly. Each new declaration of the patient's activity instigates an ever-deeper probing into the subjective dimensions of the patient's experience; each promise to honor it delivers a more precise documentation of its multiple hermeneutic contexts. A "discontinuous" history of a body of research predicated on "reformative" gestures such as these requires the genealogist to emphasize the continuity of approaches that purport to liberate the patient. After all, it is precisely in terms of agency that the patient is rendered problematic at all. While the subjective patient is, in this sense, a relatively recent invention, his or her subjectivity is the *object* of these clinical and human sciences. The patient's activity is constituted all the better to discipline it. What is clear is that the "self" of self-administration, unlike the personally medicating consumer of the nineteenth century, bears a crucial relation to the edicts of medicine. It is in terms of this relation that the patient becomes visible. To put this another way, the patient's agency becomes interesting to the extent that it deviates from what is prescribed. Indeed, it is precisely through his or her agency that the patient is rendered governable.

By the end of the twentieth century the discourse of compliance begins to dissolve into notions of autonomous selfhood and contractual individuality. In a report from 1997, the Royal Pharmaceutical Society of Great Britain argued that compliance can only come about by "a fundamental shift in the balance of power in the clinical encounter."[39] It proposed that *compliance* be replaced by the term *concordance*. "The price of compliance was dependency. The price of concordance is greater responsibility—of the doctor, for the quality of the diagnosis, the treatment and the explanation; of the patient, for the consequences of his or her choices."[40] Casting compliance as a situation in which the patient's "health beliefs" are forced to submit to the doctor's "solution," the report outlines "concordance" as follows:

> The clinical encounter is concerned with two sets of contrasted but equally cogent health beliefs—that of the patient and that of the doctor. The task of the patient is to convey his or her health beliefs to the doctor; and of the doctor, to enable this to happen. The task of the doctor or other prescriber is to convey his or her (professionally informed) health beliefs to the patient; and of the patient, to entertain these. The intention is to assist the patient to make as informed a choice as possible. . . . *Although reciprocal this is an alliance in which the most important determinations are agreed to be those that are made by the patient.*[41] (original emphasis)

The situation is perfect. No longer an effect of history or power, "health beliefs" become a personal property which the doctor need not engage so much as "respect." Nice relations are put before health gains. Under the guise of liberal empowerment, the patient leaves the clinic as a consumer—health beliefs intact, public claims on medicine diminished, options for other forms of action circumscribed, and individuality enforced.

Doctor as Drug

In one of the canonical texts of British "whole person" medicine, an analogy appears that anticipates the evocativeness of drugs for emerging rationalities of personhood and government. "By far the most frequently used drug in general practice [is] the doctor himself," it states.[42] Lamenting the fact that "no guidance whatever is contained in any text book as to the dosage in which the doctor should prescribe himself, in what form, how frequently, what his curative and maintenance doses should be," Michael Balint describes his psychoanalytic analysis of the doctor-patient relation as a "pharmacology of the drug 'doctor.'"[43]

The Doctor, His Patient and the Illness reflects the emphasis on communication in the medical literature that emerged in postwar Britain. The literature stressed the importance of the doctor-patient relation and the role of reassuring patients. The nature of the relationship between doctor and patient was thought to contribute directly to patients' satisfaction and health. This tradition sought to recognize and account for a basic margin of subjectivity in all processes of diagnosis and treatment,[44] eliciting a gaze that went beyond the patient's unique circumstances to encompass the doctor's specific effects on the patient. Doctors were trained to monitor themselves and, in turn, instill good habits of self-surveillance in their patients. This emphasis on the doctor's practical reflexivity was bound up within the notion that an important part of diagnosis and treatment was the supportive and reassuring relationship the doctor managed to cultivate with the patient. Thus the doctor's self-governing capabilities were deemed an essential basis of the care offered to patients in periods of low autonomy and self-assurance.

These ideas were typically elaborated in case studies of "what was probably the most prominent figure of pathology symbolized within this rationality; the depressed or anxious woman."[45] Here, the doctor was encouraged to "lend his confidence, in the sense of his authority, as a support to patients," in a motion that nevertheless claimed some distance from the "characteristics of rigidity, authoritarianism, and cynicism" associated with previous conceptions.[46] This gendered legacy allows us to understand this practice as a particular species of paternalism that directed attention not only to the social context of patients—their personalities—but also to the responsibility of doctors. For Balint, doctors were powerful but inherently dangerous drugs, "using themselves" on patients. The implication was that doctors "must learn reflexively to control their personalities in a self-disciplined manner."[47] Doctors were invited to make *themselves* and their "personalities" the subject of a particular sort of care and attention, and this was to form an important therapeutic mechanism. In this respect, as Thomas Osborne observes, "patient-centred medicine" envisaged a certain "doctor-centred" practice. Osborne characterizes the relation between doctor and patient in this context as one of "exemplarity."

In this tradition, "clinical experience guided the choice of treatment: a drug that 'worked' in clinical practice was an 'effective' treatment."[48] While this allowed a level of partiality about the effectiveness of a given treatment, it also turned clinical attention to the specific experience of treatment undergone by the patient—and the quality and attributes of the relation that conveyed it. Thus an important aspect of the treatment process was discussion of effectiveness and adverse effects, the idea being that the treatment was gradually titrated to the singular circumstances of the patient.

While to the contemporary sensibility these practices of doctoring may seem too subjective, too discretionary, too risky, to be entirely reliable, they expose a site of government that is all but ignored in the increasingly formalized literature on compliance. What they reveal is that the patient is not the only possible target of this problematization, but the practices of medicine as well.[49] In 1975 Irwin Rosenstock wrote in the *Journal of the American Medical Association* (*JAMA*) that proper diagnosis and treatment constitutes only half the doctor's task. "The other half, of equal importance, concerns the extent to which the patient complies with his recommendations."[50] The doctor has not "completely discharged his responsibility unless . . . he does all in his power to assure that the patient will possess the beliefs and knowledge necessary to follow his advice."[51] Made at the time that compliance begins to lodge itself as an established area of study in the United States, it may come as a surprise that this statement of doctors' responsibility augurs the dispersion of the doctor as a node of government. "The task of communication and education may be delegated to others," Rosenstock concedes, making reference to the increasing use of nurse practitioners, physician assistants, and other allied health personnel, "but," he insists, "the ultimate responsibility falls on the physician."[52] Meanwhile in Britain the practice of "whole person" care had endured certain changes. In the second edition of *The Doctor-Patient Relationship*, Kevin Browne and Paul Freeling refer to it as "a fashionable cliché," observing, "to provide whole person care the general practitioner must co-operate with a wide range of other workers, such as community nurses, health visitors and social workers," remarking, "the team approach is all the rage."[53] Resisting the overzealous use of the "team approach," they invoke Balint's emphasis on the centrality of the doctor-patient relationship to argue instead for "whole problem care."

What these statements indicate is that by the mid-1970s much of the responsibility for compliance was being offloaded to the experts of the various human sciences. If clinical thought had been aware of the active patient for some time, it is only at this point that the theories of the self promoted by the human sciences—and particularly the "psy disciplines"

—intensify the study of "self-administration." Not entirely comfortable as a responsibility of medicine, compliance is remarkable for its success in enrolling these disciplines in the task of analyzing the correspondence of patient activity with medical prescription. "Self-administration" appears so forcefully in the postwar period precisely because the self becomes visible at the nexus of medicine and the psychological sciences. If "default" impelled clinicians to think about how they gave instructions, compliance enlists a smorgasbord of experts to help explain and assist patients in the activity of aligning their behavior with medical advice. Where the formal discourse of compliance takes hold, the emphasis on doctors' reflexivity diminishes. Counseling, emotional role-playing, treatment for depression, occupational therapy, telephone help-lines, social work, nursing, as well as population strategies, such as health promotion and social marketing, are enrolled in the government of the patient. These offer themselves as means through which autonomous individuals might modify their behavior to attain a state of health both prescribed and desired. What they share is an account of noncompliance as a feature of the self—as administered by the patient.

It is in this context that we can situate the work of Sackett and Haynes, with which I began this chapter. Based at McMaster University in Canada, their efforts to formalize the definition and classificatory criteria for compliance were located within a broader episteme that sought so-called authoritative solutions to clinical problems and the consolidation of a certain type of medical authority and professional autonomy. But unlike the authority attained by the self-reflexive doctor, this stance purported to be based in an objective knowledge of drugs and treatment, in which it was not the experience of the clinic, but "objective" evidence from clinical trials that authorized the doctor's practice. This tradition, which became known as "evidence-based medicine," boasted its own scientific method, the randomized controlled trial, which quickly became the gold standard of drug evaluation.[54] While the effects of some drugs can be adequately assessed through clinical experience, the controlled trial promised to take the subjective elements out of clinical decision-making, contributing to the explosion in pharmaceutical production by making it possible to evaluate drugs with "more marginal, or less rapid effects."[55] The controlled trial "came to form the apex of a new hierarchy of medical knowledge that celebrated the weight of scientific evidence for or against a clinical intervention."[56] It served to boost the authority and professional autonomy of medicine by promising an objective knowledge of drugs.

The formal study of compliance can be placed in this context: the pursuit of "authoritative" solutions to clinical problems, and the consolidation of a certain form of evidential authority. But where patient-centered medicine placed emphasis on the reflexive cultivation of a style of doctoring as the basis for authority and care, evidence-based medicine anticipated a shift in doctor learning, such that informing oneself of the published scientific research formed the explicit goal of professional improvement. This pedagogy was to be disseminated through "formalised tools such as audits, clinical guidelines, and protocols."[57] The prioritization of this type of evidence also shaped the disciplined terms of compliance research. Sackett and Haynes favored the controlled trial method, for example, to assess interventions aimed at ensuring compliance, assuming a critical moment of change in human practice directly analogous to a drug.[58] What was also assumed here was that doctors' recommendations should invariably be followed, based as they were on "objective" scientific research. In this conception of clinical practice, it was not the nature or dynamic of the clinical relation that formed the substance upon which doctor and patient were to work, but the *behavior* of the patient, or the attributes of the regimen, that were to be changed, by means of interventions whose efficacy was best determined in abstract and specifically controlled conditions. These conditions validated in turn a specific type of intervention. Those that met with the most demonstrable success barely operated in the terrain of subjectivity at all, but were implications for product design, such as the simplification of dosing schedules. Among techniques directed at the patient, and for all the elegance of social psychological explanations, "crude" behavioral techniques had the most verifiable success within this regime of evidence. These ranged from the apparently innocuous (telephone reminders, dosing charts and calendars, alarm bells and beepers) to the heavy duty (continuous and comprehensive care, directly observed therapy, isolation orders).[59] It was rare meanwhile that the actions of prescribers were subject to the same standards of evaluation.

What emerges in the last quarter of the twentieth century then are two parallel and alternating doctrines of clinical practice that propose different models for the government of drugs and that envision different exercises of medical authority. The first, a "patient-centered medicine," grounded prescribing in patients' personal characteristics and idiosyncratic needs, with clinical experience guiding the choice of treatment and an emphasis on the doctor-patient relation. Diagnosis and treatment was a matter of collaboration—albeit uneven—between doctor and patient in the private space of the clinic. Recognizing a level of subjectivity, contingency, and variability in clinical practice, it sought to account for this by encouraging doctors to think of themselves as drugs—to exercise a disciplined self-reflexivity that would function as a model for patients in an "exemplary" sort of way. The second, "evidence-based medicine," accounted for this fallibility differently—by seeking to accumulate an objective knowledge of drugs that promised authoritative solutions to clinical problems. It proposed a method—the randomized controlled trial—as the gold standard of knowledge about interventions and reified it as the only way to gain true knowledge about drugs.[60] Because the solutions it generated were reified as objective, the extent to which patients would carry them out became the problem of government that drugs posed. Even the interventions made to ensure the proper administration of these interventions were to be evaluated as though they were drugs. This was the study of compliance.

But what sort of interventions does the controlled trial endorse? The method of evaluating a drug against a predefined outcome by delivering it to a randomized half of a patient group, with the other half receiving a placebo, renders the "effects" of the drug in a specific way. In particular, at least some of the drug's effects get consigned to the status of side effects or adverse events, with the professionally defined objective of the drug forming the privileged measure of its evaluation. The "use" of the drug is thus confined to its professionally determined objective, with other effects receding in importance. If effectiveness is understood as "the impact an intervention achieves in the real world, under resource constraints, in entire populations" and efficacy as "the improvement in health outcome achieved in a research setting, in expert hands, under ideal conditions,"[61] evidence-based medicine might be regarded as replacing the specific and multi-varied effects of drugs with a fetishized emphasis on efficacy, whose idealized conditions the patient then becomes responsible for reproducing. Compliance measures the adherence of patients to a certain configuration of knowledge and power at the expense, perhaps, of promoting the participation of specific consuming bodies in the production and contestation of health priorities and bodily realities.

A drug is not a thing—or not only. Its safety and specific effects vary according to complex assemblages of composition, interaction, timing, conduct, history, digestion, inscription, and communication. The anxieties about drug use traced in this chapter were far from groundless: the new compounds flowing from the pharmaceutical industry were efficacious only in specific conditions—with otherwise redundant, and sometimes dangerous, consequences.[62] While these facts may be used to naturalize a concern for compliance, the questions of how this problem gets framed, by whom, and with what implications for which social actors—and how this in turn authorizes some players and not others, and affects given relations of power, credibility, and production—should be emphasized. The two doctrines of medical practice outlined here distribute these elements different ways, with different implications for the authority of consumers. Neither is free from the exercise of power: they anticipate different practices of evaluation, self-relation, and negotiation.

Incorporating Clinical Authority

What are we to make of the ever-advancing disciplinary gaze? This creeping medical *and* psychological *and* sociological gaze? For, if there were any doubt, this history should disabuse us of the notion that medicine is alone in the regulation of identity. What does this account suggest for those who work in the field of health, who are concerned with the control of diseases, drugs, and epidemics, but who wish to attune themselves to, and where possible resist, the disciplinary effects of the human sciences?

I first became interested in the social regulation of drugs while investigating the topic of compliance with HIV antiretroviral treatment with colleagues at the National Centre in HIV Social Research in Sydney. When I joined the sector in 1997, the overriding question in the field was, why isn't everyone availing themselves of these new, very effective therapies? Early intervention was the order of the day, and those who were not "hitting hard and early" were viewed as a problem for education, medicine, and social research. This view, often expressed with the best of intentions and utmost concern, structured the *will to knowledge* that governed treatment research at the time, by which I mean the overarching impulse or desire that brought the research into being and motivated it. This will to knowledge governs many things, including the methods one employs, the sorts of questions one asks of the data, the aspects that are deemed significant, the form the analysis takes. In crude and perhaps overly simplistic terms, this meant that the practices and understandings of the research subjects *not on* treatment were viewed as interesting—a matter for further analysis and humane concern—while those *using treatment properly* were seen as less problematic or interesting. The discourses that shaped how social research took place in the sector had to do with the governmental investment in research as a form of expertise on health behavior. One went out into the field to collect *data*, from which one would develop an account of *unmedical behavior*, which might then be used by practitioners in the field in efforts to *change behavior*. Because the sector was well attuned to the temporality of urgency, the more that research could point to practical interventions in this regard, the more useful it was likely to be.

In the course of our research, we found that adhering to treatments was not simply viewed as a challenge, an inconvenience, or a medical necessity related to the efficacy of the drugs.[63] For at least some of the people who prescribed and were prescribed these treatments, compliance was the basis of a curious sense of moral satisfaction—a minor testament to personal virtue and self-control.[64] Given the rigors of the average dosing schedule, the widespread experience of side effects, and the years of medical insufficiency in the face of AIDS, it was not surprising that the capacity to take these regimes induced a heightened sense of relief and accomplishment. But this enthusiasm often took on an extra degree of fervor—the sort of ostentation and pride you are as likely to encounter in a fitness fanatic or aerobics instructor, whose body seems devoted to the militant demonstration of personal economy—a sort of cheerleader approach to health maintenance. Through the optic of HIV treatment compliance, this did not seem such a problem. Indeed, it was an attitude positively encouraged by the apparatus of social marketing campaigns, doctors' advice, drug company education programs, and research findings (our own included) in circulation at the time. The doctrine of "taking charge" was the order of the day, and HIV educators did their best to rally enthusiasm. But for the many HIV-positive people living on pensions or out of savings, who had lost most of their friends to the epidemic, or who had left the workforce some time ago in preparation for a death whose only grim reassurance was its character of predictability, the message was exacerbating. Many of these people found themselves trying to adjust to this mantra in such a way that the associated difficulties only ever seemed capable of materializing as a matter of personal failure, deserving of self-blame. Others found themselves on the receiving end of a cool hostility when they voiced their difficulties regarding treatment—not least from those having better luck in this regard. To make matters worse, the treatments were associated with a range of noxious physical effects including diarrhea, nausea, high blood pressure, liver damage, insomnia, fatigue, hallucinations, depression, memory problems, and other irreversible and unknown dangers. Perhaps most unexpected and distressing for many was a side effect known as lipodystrophy, a condition that comprises substantial wasting of the face, arms, legs, and buttocks and an accumulation of fat in other parts of the body.

If HIV diagnostic testing had created the possibility of being diagnosed as sick while feeling relatively healthy, viral load monitoring created the possibility of being diagnosed as acceptably healthy while feeling very unwell. Research participants conveyed the paradox of this situation: "My feeling of wellbeing is shithouse. Um, really bad. Um, actual health—like going to the doctors—is fabulous. There's a nice contradiction for you. I feel awful but my actual health is very, very good."[65] Treatment produced tensions, sometimes dire, between various measures and evaluations of living well. But according to the logic of compliance, these "side" effects were of a secondary nature, most appropriately endured and subjected to the primary goal of viral suppression.[66] The quotidian pressure of this discourse was manifest in the offhand descriptions of patients by clinicians as "good compliers" for having stuck to therapy despite a range of incapacitating effects,[67] the habitual dismissal of lipodystrophy as a legitimate concern on the basis that its effects were merely "cosmetic" (or an aspect of "lifestyle"), and the reluctance of some patients to mention to doctors the experience of treatment sicknesses on the assumption that they were an inevitable part of treatment.[68] For at least some people, the discourse of compliance seemed to evince a commitment to medicine far greater than the medical merits. Meanwhile, the results of viral load tests, when undetectable, were commonly announced as though they indicated not just the efficacy of the prescribed treatment—a reduced rate of viral replication in plasma—but were also a measure of personal worth, the amount of viral RNA circulating in the bloodstream bearing an inverse relation to the exact degree of all-round personal competence and moral accomplishment. It was as though the viral load test had taken on some localized aspects of the discursive function that Foucault attributed to sexuality, forming a new and corporeal site for revealing the truth about the self. The most excruciating aspect of this discourse was the implication that patients were to endure a range of harmful physical effects and be commended for doing so, that their capacity to dismiss what was happening to their bodies was to be valued and taken as evidence of personal prudence, responsibility, and valiant determination, and that we—researchers, educators, clinicians, health promoters—were to assist and through various means instruct them how to do so. It was our job to beget an oddly impervious pleasure consuming medicine.

A curious thing happened over the course of doing this research. The clinical guidelines completely changed. The experience of the drugs, including the development of viral resistance, the prevalence of side effects, and the existence of unforeseen long-term effects, forced a revision of treatment guidelines such that they advocated a much later intervention with treatment—some scientists even recommending postponing it until the onset of clinical symptoms.[69] What had at one moment been an imposing norm of patient behavior and clinical conduct—taken seriously enough to mobilize significant research, policy, educational, and emotional resources—was now scientifically inadvisable. There is another story to tell about how this came to be the case—about the role of clinical experience, patient accounts, and clinical counterpublics in the identification and legitimation of the experience of certain side effects and thus the *production* of scientific knowledge—but for our purposes this meant that the only "useful" parts of our research, the only parts that were in any way "practicable," were those that were not so tightly structured by the will to knowledge (concerning noncompliance). What was valuable about these data, in other words, were not the sociological and psychological explanations of noncompliance they afforded—the ability to force them into shape to fit the problematic of compliance—but rather the partial insights they gave into the material circumstances with which people with HIV were themselves engaged: how they were negotiating the difficulties of HIV illness in the context of the discursive pressures of compliance, and with what different effects. And this was important not because it made it possible to bend embodied subjects to some prior or assumed health imperative, but because they could be used as accounts to enable different agencies, including people on drugs, clinicians, and research institutions, to work together better and with attention to situated difference. This was not all. The experience also called for a critical and historical perspective on our own knowledge practices—the nature and bases of the problems we posed, the social and institutional relations that shaped the sorts of questions we asked—because we were intimately involved, often in unforeseen and absurd ways, in the sometimes unpleasant and usually inadvertent production of people's realities. In short, it was necessary to bring the historical and situated character and investments of our own "objective" gaze into the picture—to bring some attention to the disciplinary effects of social, as well as medical, science.[70] In the last three chapters of this book, I explore some embodied attempts to navigate such disciplinary conditions.

3

RECREATIONAL STATES

• • •

In the previous chapter I traced the emergence of a new form of discipline centered on the use of medicines. Through a discourse on the use and misuse of drugs, we saw how medicine becomes concerned with questions of "self-administration." In this chapter I examine the simultaneous appearance of another, similar discourse of drug misuse, this time finding expression in a different part of the social apparatus, namely the law. And I want to suggest that the appearance of medicine as a reference for self-conduct in this context represents a special investment in medical authority on the part of the state, as well as a novel function for the legal apparatus that instates it. This function corresponds with, but also seeks to suspend, broad shifts in the government of pleasure taking place at this time, giving rise to a particular expression of state authority, which can be described as "exemplary power." Exemplary power enables the state to engage citizens in terms of their normative mode of existence—consumer self-fashioning—but in a way that seeks to subject such activity by allowing the state to make of it, in certain conditions and under certain circumstances, a bad example.

One objective of this chapter, then, is to place drug legislation in the context of broader shifts taking place in the legal regulation of "illicit" pleasure in many Western jurisdictions in the postwar period. These shifts, which change the legal status of activities such as contraception, divorce, abortion, homosexuality, pornography, gambling, prostitution, and various forms of recreation, have been read as attempts on the part of the state to gear its legal apparatus to a consumer economy.[1] In some respects, these reforms are indicative of the growing influence of medicine in the treatment of "moral deviance"—an apparent softening of social attitudes, whereby many problems previously considered criminal are reconfigured as social problems, inspiring therapeutic rather than punitive attention. But they also represent the simultaneous (and somewhat contradictory) propulsion of medicine into a *juridical* role, in which medicine takes on the symbolic and political role of social order and moral control, expressed, when advantageous, through the punitive mechanisms of the law. These investments converge most forcefully in the legal construction of "drug abuse," which, through high-profile practices of patrol and reportage, is liable to manifest as an offensive example of self-administration.

At stake then is the significance of the state's stance on illicit drugs for circumscribing and defining legitimate modes of consumer citizenship. I am especially interested in the signification of drugs for consumer culture—how, within this context, they can come to embody the antithesis of the proper administration of the self. By consumer culture I mean something historically specific and economically contingent: the dense material culture to which the expansion of commodity production in the last century has given rise, encompassing advertising and mass media, and in which consumption—its sites, practices, and identities—has taken on major symbolic centrality. One feature of this context is a partial dislocation of capitalist ideology away from a Puritan ethic of hard work, accumulation, and restraint, and toward a provisional articulation around expressive, erotic, and experiential pleasures.[2] This dislocation raises certain problems for government—not least, how to contain and moderate between the conditions of licensed pleasure and disciplined productivity: how to maintain suitably encapsulated pleasures, if you like. I suggest that drugs are constructed as a sign and instance of *excessive conformity* to contemporary consumer culture—and that this excess is opportunistically scooped off and spectacularized in order to stage an intense but superficial battle between the amoral market and the moral state. The main causalities of this battle are almost always marked in terms of race, class, sexuality, gender, and citizenship status: whether incarcerated or excluded in various ways from any sort of hopeful participation in formal economies of employment or desire, or policed by sniffer dogs in their recreational precincts.[3] The "exemplary" nature of drug control enables the state to selectively exert its authority in a context where it also depends, for the generation of economic value, on a degree of free-floating social experimentation and cultural recreation.

Stan's Future Self

The story of Stan's "Future Self" gives some initial clues as to how, in the present imagination of virtuous consumer citizenship, an authoritarian stance on drugs is employed to beget order and hard work from the potentially boundless distractions of consumer recreation. In a 2002 episode of *South Park*, Stan's Future Self turns up inexplicably one day.[4] Stan is a regular kid, one of the fourth graders who comprise the main characters in this cartoon about life in a small Colorado town. One day a strange man claiming to be his Future Self turns up on the family doorstep. Appearing first on the TV news, running wildly through the town, the Future Self arrives at Stan's house, alone and disheveled, bearing pitiable tales of junkie-dom—a life ruined by drugs. At first it seems young Stan must confront the loser he will become. But as it turns out over the course of the episode, Stan's parents have hired an actor to play this future version of Stan from a company called Motivation Corp. The idea is to scare young Stan into a proper regard for his future by representing in the present a shocking projection of what it could be. In a covert operation of parental concern, the embodied spectacle of drugs is employed to dramatize the need for a personal state of enterprise among the young.

How and what do drugs embody in this underhand and precautionary deployment of becoming? To pursue this inquiry, I find myself embarking on my own excursions through time—not to a future I can preempt in a fearful defensive maneuver but to a past I will assemble in a tentative and provisional style—to explain how such an idea of the future could arise. *South Park* has a keen eye for what a certain discourse on drugs *does*—how, that is, it is exercised in the body of everyday statements. In ways that appear as cynical and manipulative, a moral stance on drugs is adopted to motivate a particular subjective disposition, entailing a particular orientation to the future and a certain ethic of existence: forward-looking, calculative, prudent, aspirational—a subject with a very precise concern for the self.[5] In linking any hope of a dignified future to individual acts of determination, continence, social compliance, and self-control, the dopey Future Self isolates the present from consideration of the conditions of labor, belonging, or public life. My aim is to show how a medico-moral discourse on drugs operates to bring this ethic of existence into being. That the misfortune attending the situated consumption of some substances is available as a horrific spectacle is not such a surprise—but what are the histories and components of this conception of wasted life? How do the multiple and diverse instances designated by the term *drugs* become comprehensible in terms of a cautionary inducement to personal enterprise and industriousness? On what basis are they assumed to motivate a subject whose conduct and future is an object of precise individual control and preemptive action? What is the nature of the investment in this subject? And why is a Future Self the particular vehicle through which its promise materializes?

A preliminary answer to some of these questions comes in the form of the emergent symbolism of drugs in the context of their increasing popularity among middle-class youth in the United States, Britain, and elsewhere from the 1960s. The case of cannabis is illustrative. In the 1930s, marijuana had the reputation of the "killer weed" in North America, based on its association with Mexican migrants and their association, in turn, with abject violence and criminality.[6] Marijuana was thought to produce a failure of restraint, stimulating aggression and leading to assault, murder, rape, or self-destruction. These properties helped justify its inclusion within existing criteria of prohibition, which rested on the concepts of narcotics and dangerous drugs. But marijuana's expanding popularity in the 1960s among a different class of users—middle-class youth and the counterculture—constituted its effects quite differently (though no less prohibitively) as the "drop-out drug." Where earlier marijuana had been associated with violence, it was now ascribed virtually opposite qualities: an apparent source of passivity and "amotivational syndrome."[7] In a protean and nebulous maneuver, the pharmacology of the drug had transformed to suit the anxiety converging on its users.

It would be easy to read this as a case of antiquated and culturally prejudiced perceptions giving way to the objective precision of modern science, but this would be to suppose that some transparent, culturally-stripped access to the problem is possible. These constructions were not mere ideology, awaiting the enlightenment of value-neutral medicine; they were not just cultural scuttlebutt. Suppose that, to Southern landholders in the 1930s, and those they rallied to define the problem, marijuana *really was* part of a problem of crime and violence committed by an oppressed Mexican laboring underclass. And that to Middle America in the 1960s, and the scientific and official players who synthesized their concerns, marijuana *really was* a problem of lack of ambition, failure to achieve, and the rejection of conventional values among their young. The coordinates of the official gaze framed how the drug's effects were apprehended and perceived. And the problem shifted according to the social situation of, and expectations converging around, its users. It is unlikely, for example, that "lack of ambition" among migrant workers was a pressing concern for the medical professionals, public officials, and law-keepers who publicized the effects of marijuana in the 1930s.[8] But it was a worrying preoccupation in regard to middle-class youth of the 1960s. And while it is impossible to determine whether marijuana "really did" induce violence on the part of migrant workers at that point in history, it is unlikely that these laboring classes were ever allowed to formulate the problem of their circumstances in terms that had a chance of being treated as legitimate, and thus reframe the situation. In these moments, the government of social tensions gets condensed into the problematization of a substance thought to be productive or indicative of them, the drug becoming a fetishized sign of that which is seen as most threatening or worrying about a situation on the part of those authorized to define it as a problem.[9] But this is not to suggest that drugs did not *do* things in bodies: they had effects, perhaps even harmful effects. And what was found interesting and problematic and harmful about these— what was determined causative about the situation and thus actionable —was a matter and function of politics: of how the technical problem was posed, and by whom.[10]

While the desire to identify something as biological and substantial to account for, supervise, and eliminate troublesome behavior was a familiar impulse at the time of early drug legislation, there were subtle differences in the drug problem that consolidated in the 1970s, partly in response to the counterculture. If habitués of narcotics were thought to be held in thrall by the intrinsic scientific and addictive properties of particular substances, there was a distinct air of defiance about the drug user of the 1960s—a sense of deliberate dissent. The increasing use of medical and other drugs for various purposes, including a simple desire for pleasure, was identified by many with a broader culture of social experimentation.[11] It was not so much the physical dangers of use, but the social symbolism of drug consumption, "the way in which it had come to represent nonconformity in general," that encapsulated official fears at this time.[12] This is not to say that theories of addiction declined in influence—far from it. As Eve Sedgwick and others have observed, they penetrated further and further into all manner of activity of everyday life.[13] But as though to emphasize the social and moral noncompliance of the (otherwise "normal") selves administering them, the legal framing of drugs transforms at this time from a concept of narcotics (and inherent physical danger) to a paradigm of misuse and abuse.

The extent of this shift is widespread, hastened by the international (if U.S.-dominated) nature of the instruments and institutions targeting the drug issue around the world. Sections of the U.S. Code previously referring to "narcotics" are renamed the *Drug Abuse Prevention and Control Act* in 1970. In the United Kingdom the *Dangerous Drugs Act* of 1920 is replaced by the *Misuse of Drugs Act* of 1971. Commissions conducted in Canada and South Australia at this time take the "Non-Medical Use of Drugs" as their focus, with Australian state legislation adopting the terminology of "misuse" in the 1980s. Where previously legislation had located the problem of drugs in the intrinsic nature of the substances proscribed—employing the language of "narcotics," for example, to group often unlike substances (heroin, cocaine, marijuana) under one rubric and suggest a measure of scientific legitimacy for their similar treatment—by the 1970s a new language of concern is taking shape. It is no longer the scientific properties of specific substances, nor the physical dangers arising from their consumption, but the *character* of their use, its deviation from professional authority, that forms the locus of juridical concern.[14] Drugs now precipitate a concern in the general domain of *self-conduct.*

I mean to draw out the situated character of this problem: the appearance of "promising youth" as the privileged object of antidrug discourse, the imprint of flouted conventions of middle-class ambition and achievement. And perhaps most manifest of all in this framing is the concerned subjectivity of the parent.[15] This reconfiguration of the drug problem around these concerns propels medicine into a new and apparently monumental role. As the explicit measure of legitimate conduct in regard to drugs, it takes on a much larger mandate. The discourse of compliance constituted the patient's relation to drugs in terms of "self-administration." In the discourse of drug abuse, this relation is reiterated, enshrined in law, and spread out across the social field to demarcate consumer propriety *in general*. Medicine becomes an index of social propriety, marking the parameters of normal conduct in a dogmatic iconicity of authority. But in a peculiar way, medicine is a puppet here. It is appealed to as a ground of social authority—to contest the perceived affront to established order and professional power—often *irrespective* of the physical effects of particular substances. This has unanticipated consequences. It makes it possible, for example, for a counter-discourse on "harm reduction" to emerge, taking as its aim avoidance of the more patent physical harms of drugs (often at the initiative of, or with support from, medical professionals).[16] But to reapply an earlier description, the dominant conception of drug abuse that emerges at this time spells a commitment to medicine *far greater* than the medical merits.[17] It announces a case of social deviancy that takes its very bearings from compliance with medical authority. The figure of medicine stands in here, in legal garb, to propound a standardized identity for the parent.

This brings us back to Stan's Future Self, who does not embody the outcome of a specific series of ingestive practices so much as the threat thought to be posed by such practices to a particular notion of the administration of the self—one that places a premium on a certain conception of the future rooted in white middle-class ambitions and aspirations. By impersonating these fears from the past, the Future Self compels and reproduces this image of life for the future—propagating an ethic at once enterprising and precautionary, in which the self is held responsible for the economic and ambitious possession of the body. This is life conceived as an individually managed project, in which the self is invited to realize the self, but must also assume responsibility for any excesses that this process of self-actualization occasions. There is nothing particularly wrong or invalid about this conception of life, but it does not begin to describe or explain the conditions or effects, the variable and structurated nature, the situated character of the pleasures and the dangers of the experience of drugs in society. The Future Self appears as an isolated figure. But because this image of drugs is communicated in the sensorium of fear and alerts the subjectivity of the parent, it is remarkably available for imposing this idea on a broader populace: for organizing general insecurities so that they take out insurance in this conception of life and the future.[18] Profiled in the law as crime, and implemented by global instruments in diverse jurisdictions, it is surprisingly adaptable for conjuring in diverse contexts Protestant-inspired notions of self-control and personal discipline, elaborated against a global scenography of consumer pleasure.[19] In the chapters that follow, I will offer some concrete examples of how this construction has been used to startle into existence a particular conception of the good life. But first, I want to consider in more detail how it connects with some broader ways of conceiving the possibilities of social identity and political practice that arise at this time, beginning with a consideration of some of the changes, in the Western consumer context, in the social government of pleasure.

The Government of Pleasure

The consumer context brought changes to the legal status of many activities previously considered illicit. Greater employment and the expansion of welfare after the Second World War created a new margin of freedom for citizens. The emergence of new markets targeting women and youth —particularly in terms of their capacity for self-directed pleasure and eroticized consumption—were significant features of this trend. If the rise in the social wage enabled an incipient generational consciousness and a new sphere of social freedoms, it also opened up new markets upon which the consumer economy came to rely. In many first world jurisdictions this was facilitated by important changes in the government of pleasure, with legal restrictions on pornography, contraception, abortion, divorce, homosexuality, gambling, prostitution, and various forms of recreation removed or reworked. An almost universal exception to the general trend in states' realization or implementation of an economy based on consumer pleasures was the position on illicit drugs. Here states tended to abandon the governing rationality and, as Stuart Hall writes in relation to the British context, "legislated in a thoroughly reactionary direction."[20]

In general, these reforms involved carving out a sphere of personal privacy within which "immoral"—but no longer illegal—conduct was to be contained. This was true of the law, but it also usefully describes the shift in respect of these practices in the general locus of social control.

Gambling is a good example.[21] Traditionally, opposition to working-class gambling was grounded in doctrines of Protestant morality, it being thought symptomatic of a lack of discipline and a source of social decay. Legislative attempts to prohibit and regulate gambling over the course of the twentieth century met with little success. But a gradual redefinition of gambling as a form of entertainment and leisure for which people paid—a "pleasurable commodity" (and a business) rather than a vice—justified its reform and legalization at this time according to the terms of neoliberal consumer culture. As a commodity, gambling could be thought regulated through the market and the free choices of individuals. It became intelligible as a legitimate consumer pleasure. Particularly interesting for our purposes though are the attempts made to reconfigure the problematic personal and social aspects of gambling in this context. While notions of illness had long been a part of antigambling discourses, these now drew on the language of "compulsion" and "addiction" to describe the unwanted effects of the activity. In this language, "the problem of gambling was reconceived as one of individual excess, rather than widespread social participation."[22] Problem gambling became a condition of the self.

The example of gambling makes it possible to see how medicine is implicated in the circumscription of a regime of the personal. If legal prohibition represents regulation by and on behalf of a putative public, notions of addiction and therapy delegate this task to the private person, presenting it as a corollary of "healthy free will."[23] Medicine draws a circle around the individual subject of consumption, with the notion of "addiction" acting as a sort of drawstring. But what is the significance of the state's grasp on illicit drugs? What sort of place does it organize for the state in the oscillation of incitement and control, the play of liberation and restraint, that characterizes the consumer context? To really grasp its full significance here, we need to consider just how mundane drugs are in terms of the sorts of pleasures animated in this setting. Many authors have noted the utility of a culture of excitement, transgression, self-expression, and romance for the purposes of modern commodity culture, with varying degrees of distaste.[24] (Indeed, it's sometimes hard to know whether it is in fact commodity culture, or the prospect of pleasure itself, that most incites these somber tomes.) Pat O'Malley and Stephen Mugford draw on these analyses to argue that, when set in a context where experiential novelty designates the attraction of many goods and services (including some dangerous forms), the recreational practice of drugs appears "an intelligible form of the normatively sanctioned search for the extraordinary."[25] They point to the values of exploration, novelty, intensity, longing, excitement, self-expression, hedonism, and imagination commonly transmitted in this setting. When considered in this light, the species of private hedonistic pleasure that drugs embody, far from being an anathema to the conservative face of economic liberalism, appears as a requisite of some of its most indispensable transactions.

The notion of drug use as an instance of conformity (one might say *excessive conformity*) to consumer culture runs counter to how many individuals framed their drug practice in the 1960s. But it is in this context (in which consumption establishes itself at the constitutive center of social life) that a vast proportion of drug use comes to be understood as "recreational." And while it would be incorrect entirely to paint the popular focus on expressive and experiential pleasures as some ruse of capital, it can certainly be said that capital sought to utilize and profit from it. Many forms of self-expression and exploration, previously forbidden, become permissible and even expected in this context, evoking what Mike Featherstone describes as "a calculating hedonism."[26] The consumer is invited to participate in a certain normative relaxation of emotional controls—one that allows for a greater exploration of the expressive and the experiential—but is also made responsible for reining these back in: for maintaining what Cas Wouters depicts as a "controlled de-control of the emotions."[27] And it is against this background—the contemporary correspondence of consumer pleasure and drugs—that the legal position on drugs takes on a special significance. For if drugs can be considered relatively typical as a consumer pleasure, their prohibition reserves for the state a distinct moral position in the field of pleasure. Further, it refers any responsibility for the casualties of consumption back onto the consuming self. Where the notion of addiction draws a circle around the subject of consumer pleasures, the concept of abuse reinforces it with the heavy machinery of the law, operating now as the *hard edge* of this deployment of medical authority. And as the stopping point of permissive legislation, drug law gains the capacity to conjure up a moral state—suggesting, if only fleetingly, the possibility of an alignment between state command and the contents of that space carved out for personal variation. It instates as its vision of control a regime of the personal—installing the self as the medium of liberation *and* control.

If the domain of the personal was the primary beneficiary of the relative prosperity of the postwar period, in conditions of world recession it was increasingly constructed as precisely the object according to whose control order was to be maintained.[28] In this context the ground of social authority offered by medicine under the sign of drugs becomes particularly enticing for power. Experts and politicians often make a (very practicable) distinction between medical and criminal approaches to drug use, but perhaps this distinction misunderstands the broader political and economic forces that invest this site.[29] It is not a rational preference for medical or criminal approaches that accounts for the selection of strategies at a given juncture, but the *political investment in self-administration as a node of social control*. Power never knows whether it wants to punish or save the drug user, incarcerate or treat this figure. Instead, both strategies are kept in reserve as mutually reinforcing alternatives. It is almost always the underprivileged—those marked by class or race—that bear the brunt of the sterner form of discipline. Meanwhile, if not electing rehabilitation and treatment for themselves, the more privileged are ushered in its general direction in concerned but insistent tones. So long as medicine remains the parental monitor of recreational activity, the trope of self-administration is available to be more or less severely enforced. In periods of socioeconomic unrest, it is ready to find a more severe expression in an authoritarian performance of drug control, converting generalized instability into a matter of personal regimes.

In this sense medical authority marks the site of a certain becoming-conservative of consumer culture. And there is something very interesting in this phenomenon, because, as I have said, medicine is a puppet here. It is doing the work of public order and social control, and it is doing it in a symbolic register. Thus it consistently seeks the value of publicity: to attain a public significance. There are interesting parallels with the broader symbolism of health in the cultural landscape at this time. Robert Crawford has described the health and fitness craze in America from the 1970s as one in which "middle-class identity and self-control is secured and conspicuously displayed."[30] Perhaps this is where compliance finds its authoritarian expression: as a volitional intensity at the level of the person. Appropriately, perhaps, the discourse that takes the active patient as its object is embraced with exemplary activity. The performance of health is pursued here not simply for the purposes of achieving health, but in order to *express* certain values—"self-control, self-discipline, self-denial, will power."[31] A personal morality converging around the body claims public relevance and consequence, the body forming the site of a spectacular demonstration of personal economy. Out of the rubble of the welfare state springs the vigorous figure of the health consumer, still inspired by the themes of self-determination and the personal-as-political, but now embracing the discipline of the active subject in a visceral enthusiasm for health, efficiency, and independence —a body at once liberated *and* conservative, exuding recreation *and* productivity.

How might we think about this instantiation of a medical authority? A performance that makes on behalf of sovereignty a spectacle of the non-medical administration of bodies? I want to characterize it here as *exemplary power*. Consumer culture is generally understood in terms of the operation of "soft" forms of surveillance, in which autonomous citizens regulate themselves through organizing their lives around the market, allowing disciplinary and welfare technologies to be downscaled. In these terms, drug control might be considered one of the "harder" puni-tive and behavioral mechanisms that are said to flank these "softer" technologies of social control. But this would be to miss the declarative character of this exercise of power, its operation in the vicinity of indi-vidual self-fashioning and display. It would not quite capture the way it engages the technologies of pleasurable consumption, or takes advantage of the techniques through which the concept of the public testing of the private self is gradually embedded in consciousness.[32] The spectacular character of drug control represents a specific combination of powers, of particular utility to the conservative recreational state. It is an *exemplary* (rather than merely disciplinary) form of power. It exemplifies the state's propensity to instate regimes of self-administration. It relies on high-profile media and police presence, making of certain practices of cultural consumption a bad example. The sample and the moral example are its favorite tools—the sample claiming to measure objectively the extent to which an individual has complied with medico-moral regimes—making a biochemical example of the propriety of individual behavior.[33] Exemplary power marks the bounds of legitimate consumer citizenship by declaring a stop to (what it designates as) nonmedical activity. It is haunted by the memory of a discipline at once paternalistic and protective, which it seeks to supplant by instating as its vision of control a medico-moral imagery of the self.

Using Culture

Having sketched the particular investment in drugs that arises in this context, I now want to consider some of the critical and theoretical approaches that have attempted to respond to the totalizing force of consumer culture. It soon becomes clear that a tropography of drugs runs through these approaches. When introducing the possibility of an active, critical consumption of popular culture, for example, Stuart Hall writes:

> Now, if the forms and relationships, on which participation in this commercially provided "culture" depend, are purely manipulative and debased, then the people who consume and enjoy them must either be themselves debased by these activities or else living in a permanent state of "false consciousness." They must be "cultural dopes" who can't tell that what they are being fed is an updated form of the opium of the people. That judgment may make us feel right, decent and self-satisfied about our denunciations of the agents of mass-manipulation and deception—the capitalist cultural industries: but I don't know that it is a view which can survive very long as an adequate account of cultural relationships; and even less as a socialist perspective on the culture and nature of the working class. Ultimately, the notion of the people as a purely *passive*, outline force is a deeply unsocialist perspective.[34]

Hall's influential statement of consumer agency signalled a departure from the Frankfurt School, whose depictions of individuals wrenched from their traditional and communal structures, left vulnerable to manipulation and ideological control at the hands of the mass media, dominated critical approaches to consumption until this time. The cultural dope evokes the addictive intonations of the Frankfurt perspective, which

typically presented consumer culture as compounding modern alienation by offering a realm of delusory satisfactions and identities through
the medium of the market, "false needs" that appear all the more enticing
given the breakdown of traditional ties. In this view, consumers are
depicted rather passively as uncritically accepting the ideology of capitalist production. The individualizing dreams of the market gradually re-
place communal and class-ethnic identifications, distracting individuals
from the reality of their condition and short-circuiting any possibility of
resistance. Political acquiescence is not the only prognosis in this account: the more the commodity is invested with the hope of overcoming
the alienated condition, the more human relationships are impoverished
and wrenched apart; thus the consumer is doomed to perpetual dissatis-
faction and an ongoing "re-creation of frustration."[35]

The standard response to this perspective, in British cultural studies
and American liberal sociology alike, has been "to look for the redeeming
features of commodity culture in the act of consumption . . . to find forms
of mass consumption that were not 'passive' and types of mass consumers
who were not stupefied, to provide a sociology of watching and reading
and listening."[36] Enter the cultural dope—a figure lumped with the unhappy role of embodying all that this new vision of consumer possibility
was *not*. Though Hall places considerable emphasis on the precarious
nature of the parameters of resistance thus imagined, the cultural dope
takes on a life of its own, becoming (by inversion) an identifying feature
of a body of work that celebrates the ability of individuals and groups to
"make themselves" as well as to be made by the culture of consumption.
Taking its cue from British subcultural theory, this literature figures
consumption not as a blueprint of alienation, but a site of creative and
symbolic play through which oppositional identities are forged. Consumers were not dupes who passively soaked up the messages of cultural
producers: they were actively involved in practices of symbolic creativity
that allowed new and unconventional social identities to emerge. Meaning was not fixed once and for all in consumer objects: rather it depended
on the ways these objects were taken up and used, the social practices in
which they were embedded. (Thus Hebdige's famous safety pin meant
something quite different pierced through a punk's ear than it did in
mum's haberdashery kit).[37] Consumption was not an obvious instrument
of alienation. Rather, it was being used to forge social relations, group

ethos, and status distinctions in ways marked by the social relations of class, race, and gender.

A key conceptual move in this approach entailed a shift in emphasis away from the formal determinations of the social structure and toward a consideration of the enunciative variety of lived practice. Inspired by the work of the French theorist Michel de Certeau, the question of how products were taken up and *used* becomes an issue of considerable analytic investment and political longing, the focus no longer so much on the ideological determinations of production but on the localized appropriations and inhabitations of power, the conviction being that practice and process exceeded the formal determinations of the social system. Consumption appears as itself a form of production, in the sense of a subtle and unpredictable reworking of the social order.[38] In this incarnation, cultural studies could be thought to propose a "vision of liberation via enunciative practices" (to borrow a phrase from Margaret Morse)— an emancipatory politics of use.[39]

Drugs play a marginal role in this construction of social possibility, marginal in the sense that they actually mark out its margins. Alongside the cultural dope (whose rebuke becomes so prevalent that Meaghan Morris wonders humorously if "somewhere in some English publisher's vault there is a master disk from which thousands of versions of the same article about pleasure, resistance, and the politics of consumption are being run off under different names with minor variations"[40]) gather a number of similarly abject images of less-than-sovereign consumption. British scholar Lawrence Alloway writes in 1969, "We speak for convenience about a mass audience but it is a fiction. The audience today is numerically dense and highly diversified. Just as the wholesale use of subception techniques in advertising is blocked by the different perception capacities of the members of any audience, so the mass media cannot reduce everybody to one drugged faceless consumer."[41] And in the quite different tradition of American mass-communications research, the image of the hypodermic needle is used to critique earlier approaches to mass communication (which presumed a one-directional stimulus-response model of communication). Parodying the sense of the mass media injecting harmful ideas and behavior directly into passive individuals (attributed to suspicious European and Marxist philosophers), the image of the hypodermic needle is used to effect a transition away from this image of all-powerful communication and toward a "uses and gratifications" approach, which focused on the psychological "uses" messages serve for particular individuals. The "hypodermic model" is debunked in a glowing vision of plural and divergent audiences, eminently active and empirically knowable, bearing individual and unique *uses* for messages.[42]

Appearing everywhere at the margins of a vision of activity, the drugged-out consumer plays a poignant counterpoint to conceptions of agency in the expanding force-fields of consumption and mass communication.[43] Excluded as an adequate image of consumption, it forms the abject figure against which these theories of resistance are articulated. The prevalence of this imagery at this juncture suggests a certain complicity with the operation that Eve Sedgwick has observed of addiction in consumer capitalism: the compulsion "to isolate some new, receding but absolutized space of pure voluntarity."[44] And indeed this is exactly the claim made against some versions of cultural studies; where the Frankfurt School perspective is thought to paint a grim picture of destruction by popular culture, cultural studies of pleasure and resistance have been criticized for providing too optimistic a celebration of it, in effect reproducing voluntaristic and populist accounts of liberation that sound all too suspiciously like the individualizing dreams of the market. So it doesn't seem at all improbable that the wild proliferation of addiction theories and the "thousands of articles" Morris mentions are part of the same epistemological junction. But what are the points of overlap between cultural studies and commodity culture, and how might an investigation of drugs help us identify some of the less compromised interstices of practice?

In some respects, the assimilation of cultural politics to a consumer logic may reveal nothing more than their shared conditions of possibility. As consumers, we are unique individuals with needs, identities, and lifestyles, which we express through the purchase of appropriate commodities. In Michael Warner's argument, the endless opportunities presented for the expression of personal difference rub up against the self-abstraction demanded by the traditional public sphere (which requires individuals to deny their embodied particularity in order to recognize themselves as subjects). The contradiction between self-abstraction and self-realization is thus "forced to the fore in televisual consumer culture." He observes that "the major political movements of the last half century have been oriented towards status categories. Unlike almost all previous social movements . . . they have been centrally about the personal identity formation of minoritized subjects."[45] Similarly, if we accept Simon Frith's summation that the sociological turn in mainstream cultural studies often boiled down to a reading of popular texts in which the task was to evaluate how well the text represented or expressed the identity of particular groups—"The value of cultural goods could therefore be equated with the value of the groups consuming them—youth, the working class, women" [46]—the susceptibility to a commodity logic seems even more pronounced. An analysis of how groups use commodity texts to express themselves bears a real affinity with the consumer conception of self-representation.[47] Margaret Morse draws even stronger parallels between this variety of cultural politics and the commodified culture of self-realization, proposing: "De Certeau's very means of escape are now built into the geometries of everyday life, and his figurative practices of enunciation . . . are modeled in representation itself. Could de Certeau have imagined, as he wrote on walking as an evasive strategy of self-empowerment, that there would one day be video cassettes that demonstrate how to 'power walk'?"[48]

The intimacy of identity politics and consumer culture is often used to disparage the political gains of these movements and shore up distinctly chauvinist claims. But locating identity politics' conditions of possibility in consumer culture does not diminish the gains these movements have made. While we might share Warner's sense of the limitations of identity politics, it is worth stating that the women's movement, civil rights, and gay liberation have reconfigured the status of subordinated groups and challenged the conditions of access to public goods in important (if not yet satisfactory) ways.[49] I want also to suggest that there is something worth retrieving about the emphasis on embodied pragmatics that the politics of consumption has helped to bring into focus.[50] There is a distinct problem, after all, in rejecting outright—as already assimilated by commerce—the reconfigurative aspects of enunciative practice. Little scope is left for a politics of experience or for understanding how, against the odds of mass cultural atomization, popular histories are transmitted, lived, and recognized as a basis for action and contest—and in ways that continue to pose considerable challenges to the terms of power. Paul Gilroy for example has proposed the production, circulation, and consumption of music as a model for conceiving how black histories and cultural meanings have been transmitted in a manner that exists alongside, but in a profound sense has sought to resist, the logic of commodity relations.[51] He wants to avoid the limited political alternatives of a fixed essence of identity versus a voluntaristic and apolitical constructivism (both of which seem confirmed, incidentally, as interchangeable strategies in the commoditized context that requires individuals to express, through acts of choice in the world of goods, both who they *are* and *wish to be*). For Gilroy, the ground of resistance consists in "a changing, rather than an unchanging same" rooted in "histories of borrowing, displacement, transformation and continual reinscription" that remain "the outcome of practical activity: language, gesture, bodily significations, desires."[52]

Part of the problem threading through the study of enunciative practice is that the triumph of process over structure can often end up sounding like a celebration of individual uniqueness, self-expression, and personal preference, romantically (even repetitiously) invested in the individual ingenuity and sophistication of users. The irony here is that the image of isolated consumption embodied in the cultural dope is exactly the conception of existence these studies of popular culture set out to dispute. While the "uses and gratifications" approach is shaped by a certain psychological individualism, the emphasis on use in cultural studies stems from a tradition that stresses the shared conditions of the repertoire of uses. These uses are collectively enacted, in the sense that they derive from specific social relations and mechanisms of signification and depend for their meaning on shared, albeit heterogenous, histories and systems of value. Any competence in the art of manipulating texts is an effect of shared competences and presumes a background of collective practice, sense, and expertise. So, for example, John Frow uncovers how de Certeau's "enunciative tactics" consist of practices "in which the interlacing of speaking positions weaves an oral fabric without individual owners, creations of a communication that belongs to no-one."[53] In this sense, the reduction of the concept of "use" to an individual property or innate competence mistakes the source and site of the transformations such "uses" come to effect.

The prominence here of the theme of "use" (albeit variously theorized) points to one of the key social and political identities that arises at this time, that of the "user." But it also gives some insight into the particular species of cultural regulation that goes on under the sign of drugs. For it is precisely a domain of activity called "use" that the new legal construction of drugs totalizes. As Desmond Manderson observes, citing the United Kingdom's *Misuse of Drugs Act* of 1971: " 'Misusing a drug,' [the Act] explains placidly, means 'misusing it by taking it.' There is no such thing as taking it without misusing it."[54] Where theories of popular consumption invest in various ways in a notion of differential uses (in which agency derives from the multiform uses made of mass culture), the official conception of drugs collapses all instances of use into "abuse." Here, drug abuse does not specify "abuse" as a subset in the range of uses, but abuse *as identified by* drugs. The object trumps its enunciative variety. This step invests medicine—or the authority that medicine is taken to represent—with a specific regulative significance. Specifically, it realizes the power of the state to regularize consumer conduct through a legal commentary on self-administration. By proposing a disastrous uniformity across all instances of use, drugs become spectacularly available to create a demand for authority in the field of consumption. They materialize as the dangerous terrain that warns all instances of use must be authorized. The illicit drug coalesces state power and medical authority in such a way that it forms a poignant index of the propriety of consumption. In the same move in which drugs are identified as a question of use, the capacity to distinguish between different practices of use is put into question. Or rather that capacity is arrogated by the state. This is an action, at once totalizing and individualizing, that renders the nature and consequences of consumption an entirely personal, moral property. It works by connecting the promise of sovereignty to personal acts of continence and obedience, setting up a false symmetry between recreational states, and manifesting what I have described as exemplary power.

Perhaps this is why comparatively few studies in this tradition of cultural studies take drug use itself as an explicit focus. Despite some initial entries in the volume *Resistance Through Rituals*, it has been rare until recently to find more than cursory attention devoted to the topic in the literature on pleasure and consumption.[55] This fact is especially surprising given that the darling object of these analyses, the youth subculture, is a site of apparent prevalence. But until recently, the matter of drugs has been a blind spot in this body of research. For an analytic that proposes significant distinctions between differential instances of use, the conflation of all uses as "abuse" in the official discourse on drugs may make it a particularly tricky subject. Certainly, the possibility of danger in at least some instances of use makes it an uninviting ground in which to stake an affirmative vision of consumer experimentation. (And yet it seems clear to many of those working in the drug field that an appreciation of the different circumstances of use, and their systemic dimensions, is precisely what is needed for the cultivation of sustainable ways of averting harm).[56] Whatever the reasons for this apparent lack of interest, by remaining untackled, this image of utter consumption is all too available to limit cultural hopes of resilience and transformation. Indeed, it is precisely the scope of these hopeful aspirations it is conscripted to domesticate.

At the turn of the millennium in the political culture of Australia and America, the image of the cultural dope has come back to haunt us. But now, instead of throwing into relief the transformative possibilities of a new phase of capital, it is proposed in the figure of Stan's Future Self—as a real possibility and likely scenario, advertising the possibility of "destruction by popular culture" in a bid (ironically enough) to compel adherence to privatized and acquisitive ways of being. After a long and innovative history of harm reduction in Australia, drugs have recently begun to feature in more reactionary and spectacular political formations. The theme of future security, as realized by individual moral determination and the tender exercise of authority, has become the overwhelming theme of media interventions that, as discussed in the next chapter, ironically seem bent on arousing anxiety. Suffice it to say that an acquisitive culture of self-realization found its generative other at this moment in the idea of Stan's Future Self—the cultural dope writ large. (An unlikely convergence with Frankfurt theory, to say the least.)

Margaret Morse has described everyday life in televisual consumer culture in terms of an "attenuated fiction effect" in which "dreams become habit."[57] In this respect, there is a certain perverse logic to how the image of addiction has appeared as the moral extreme and condensation point of contemporary cultural hopes and fears. But what is curious about this figure and its deployment in the present circumstances is how it channels, ever more intently, general energies into private and guarded ways of being, reiterating the self as the medium of liberation and control. Drugs are conscripted in a discursive and affective assemblage that works to keep popular culture *personal*—and thus limit its transformative possibilities. This is accomplished by amplifying the affects of fear and disgust associated with the isolated hazards of one form of consumption (drugs), and putting it to work to model—and create an anxious demand for—authoritarian techniques aimed at domesticating consumption *in general*. I understand this as a conversion of the materializations of consumption—from an *inquisitive* and connective register to an *acquisitive* and personal register. If consumption (understood as an appropriation of meanings) harbors possibilities for connective and communicative counterpractices, the sensationalization of hazardous instances remodels these impulses into defensive and subjectified desires for the property of the personal. What may become necessary at this juncture is to depersonalize and historicize such practices of the self. "As for what motivated me, it was quite simple; . . . It was curiosity—the only kind of curiosity, in any case, that is worth acting upon with any degree of obstinacy: not the curiosity that seeks to assimilate what it is proper for one to know, but that which enables one to get free of oneself."[58]

4

DRUGS AND DOMESTICITY

• • •

Fencing the Nation

If, as Michel Foucault suggested, liberalism proceeds on the suspicion that one always governs too much, it is by this principle endowed with a remarkable capacity to enlist various (and disparate) critiques and dissatisfactions with state practice to the purpose of dislodging the traditional ambit of state responsibility.[1] This process only looks like retreat. Responsibility for social risks is indeed devolved, but indirect techniques for controlling individuals are advanced, promoted in terms of a moral vocabulary of "self-care."[2] One of the challenges for a national culture disaggregating in this way is how to contain, channel, even profit from the fears, resentment, and anxiety that accompany the loss of various prior forms of security. The theme of drugs can be rallied to this purpose —inciting, concentrating, and managing the fear surrounding changes to the economic, political, racial, and sexual landscape of our time, while also refiguring expectations, demarcations, and investments in the realms of the public and the private. As the globalization of economic and cultural transactions proceeds, drugs are put to work to align the family and nation in a seductive and nostalgic imaginary that marks out and delimits horizons of personal and collective action, bearing repercussions for sex, race, and the production and distribution of material (in)security.

My thinking on this matter has been influenced by the ways drugs have recently featured in the conservative rhetoric of Australian politicians on both sides of the political fence. After a long and relatively progressive history of harm reduction in Australia, which has provided an alternative to the negative health impacts of a prohibitionist stance on users, drugs recently began to feature in more reactionary and spectacular political formations. In 2000, the Prime Minister's office took the unusual step of intervening in the production of a national drugs campaign, insisting that it reflect a more authoritarian approach by parents, and that the booklet bear the title "Our Strongest Weapon Against Drugs . . . Families."[3] The title was later modified to the slightly milder *Our Strongest Defence Against the Drug Problem . . . Families,* and the booklet was mailed, a few months before the federal election of 2001, to "every home in Australia." When one lives, as I did at the time, on a street where heroin users wheeling prams around are a fairly common sight, one has to wonder about the efficacy of this advice. (I've not yet been game enough to ask whether there are babies in those prams or whether these characters are counting on exactly the sort of presumptions informing campaigns like this to push more than just prams, but either way they appear to shoot holes in its premises.) At about this time, a word entered Australian political discourse with such force, and with such an apparent monopoly on its signification, that I found myself wondering whether I had ever understood the real sense of the term. The election, by all accounts, hinged on the voting patterns of the new "aspirational" class. *Aspiration* was taken to denote mobility—both "upward" and "outward," economic and geographic. A mortgage-holding, double-income, upwardly mobile, lower-middle class was constructed, resident in the outskirts of major cities. A creature of focus-group testing conducted in electorally significant areas on the part of both major political parties, the aspirationals were said to "believe in the private sector and in being self-reliant; they are individualistic, competitive, and materialistic; they belong to private health funds, own shares; they are heavily in debt to their mortgages, their credit cards, and their cars . . . they are, in the main, opposed to asylum seekers and migrants whom they see as a threat to what they hold dearest of all: a high standard of living."[4] The reference to asylum seekers recalls the *Tampa* affair, which saw the government intercept and turn away a boat of Afghani asylum-seekers, purportedly to great electoral effect. It became fitting, over the course of these events, to detect the drug campaign's "weapon" as the suppressed referent of the (now ubiquitous) term *defence,* and understand this affective posture as a basic component of what Paul Kelly, writing on the significance of John Howard's reelection, described as Howard's conception of national life: a "family based aspirational society."[5]

I mean to draw out the associations here between a privatized ethic of the self, a barricaded sense of domestic space, a defensive stance toward the unfamiliar, and a heteronormative conception of intimate life. But rather than suggest these amount to some characteristic set of national attributes, I want to show how they are transmitted onto and into bodies by the discursive and affective mediation of a regime of the personal. I'm inspired here by Anna Gibbs's idea that "the media act as vectors in affective epidemics in which something else is smuggled along: the attitudes and even specific ideas which tend to accompany affect in any given situation."[6] But I do not quite mean to suggest that drugs are deployed in some crude and deliberate attempt at media manipulation designed to beget "aspirationals." Rather, a historically situated and discursively loaded fear of drugs characterizes a particular worldview, and these fears and desires get embedded in quite precise and deliberate media interventions that, ultimately, are no less crude or manipulative. But just as often, they seem entirely natural and right to their proponents: the earnest reflection of real concerns and a proper way to live.

In order to apprehend this dynamic, I'll change tacks slightly and develop a reading strategy that could be described as "radical compliance." Consistent with my earlier impulse to take medico-morality at face value, I simply do as I'm told and *dope myself out* on television.[7] As I am keen to explore how U.S. nationalist themes and imagery circulate via illicit drug discourse to become available for opportunistic deployment in local political maneuvers, my archive consists of a number of drug films and media that were finding their way into VCR and DVD players and onto Australian TVs at this time—one could call it an "archive of power." The organizing logic here is partly temporal, and partly the remarkable consistency of imagery and themes across these films and Australian TV campaign material.[8] A striking feature of these media is their appeal to a certain concept of the future. If *South Park* perceptively identified the appearance of a Future Self within antidrug initiatives—a damaged figure who returns from the future to compel compliance with authorized forms of subjectivity and enterprising citizenship—I now wish to flesh out this figure and explore its assimilation of other categories such as sex, gender, race, and class. I argue that antidrug discourse has more to do with demarcating the bounds of moral citizenship than with responding to any real threat occasioned by drugs; its concern with the future represents a fearful investment in the reproduction of the same, at the expense of more careful attention to the sociomateriality of bodies. In the previous chapter, I suggested that the mobilization of antidrug morality has an expressly strategic intent and symbolic effect, which I characterized as exemplary power. I now wish to inhabit some of these narratives and luxuriate in their modeling of safety and danger, to ask the question—well, *what do they exemplify?*

Traffic: *Suspending "Face-Time" in Late Capital*

"When Americans make the pilgrimage to Washington they are trying to grasp the nation in its totality," writes Lauren Berlant. She describes this journey as a "test of citizenship competence," for "one must be capable not just of imagining, but of managing being American."[9] When *Traffic* (Steven Soderbergh, dir., 2000) shows the protagonist, Robert Wakefield, in his new office after hours, having recently taken up the public office of drug czar—the White House bulging promisingly in the moonlight through his window—it is just such a pilgrimage that he is supposed to have undertaken. After an initial preparatory visit to Washington, he returns to his family to report proudly on the prospect of doing "face-time" with the president. The president remains uncannily faceless throughout the film, but the escalating drug habit of Caroline, Wakefield's teenage daughter, comes to be hypothesized as a function of lack of "face-time" with her father. Depicting a nation fractured by the structural tensions of late capital—between work and home, public and private, and by the porosity of national borders—the remedy *Traffic* offers is to revert to a logic of familial identification, envisioned in terms of proper parenting and the reinstatement of the absent father, who in turn must appear as an authoritative but tender head of household.[10]

The film weaves together several stories with a level of complexity that can itself be interpreted as symptomatic of the fractured, confusing world it sets out to portray.[11] In an early sequence a primary theme is declared: Drug Enforcement Agency (DEA) cops chase a suspect into a children's amusement park. The threat drug trafficking poses to the world of children is announced. From the onset, *Traffic* makes an incisive and self-justified critique of the "war on drugs." But the vision of the future this critique contains expounds a brutally neoconservative version of the nation-state, in which the overriding question is how to protect the "infantile citizen" from the excesses of contemporary America.[12]

It is true the drug problem that *Traffic* depicts traverses socioeconomic, racial, and national lines. But it is not the drug problem that is properly identified with lack of economic stability and inadequate prospects of housing, jobs, or education for the underprivileged in the modern metropolis. Rather, the drug problem that *Traffic* frets about is the risk of displacement drugs are thought to pose to the vulnerable members of privileged white families. The primary engine of fascination and horror in the film is the daughter Caroline's habit, and almost all of the drug use that takes place occurs among her and her resolutely privileged peers. Caroline is a "straight-A student," and to a large extent the drama revolves around the possible derailment of her aspirations. But the sort of mobility her compulsion produces, and the type of disorientation it represents, is inscribed as more chilling than this: in a basic sense, Caroline misrecognizes home. When she visits a seedy hotel with her boyfriend to inject drugs (always a point of intense intrigue in drug films), she murmurs, as her drugs kick in, "Wish we could just stay here, just be here forever and have a room—make a little home here." The hotel is depicted grittily in a run-down, ethnically-mixed neighborhood, and this has the effect of rendering Caroline's desire both brash and pitiable, the indiscriminate indifference of adolescence. In her delirium, Caroline seems happy to trade the stability and security of home for the transience of a rented room. Later in the film Caroline escapes from the rehabilitation program that her parents have placed her in. Her father eventually finds her in a hotel room with a man who is apparently a client, after sex. After throwing the man out, he approaches Caroline, who lies in bed dazed and sleeping. She is so doped that she is oblivious to her whereabouts or what has been happening, and so is not surprised to wake and see her father. "Hi Daddy," she says dreamily, in the quintessential (but horrifically mistaken) tenor of domestic harmony, and her father breaks down in tears.

At the thematic heart of Caroline's fall from grace, then, is an apparently willful mistaking of domestic space; a misapprehension that *Traffic* treats with a pitying and anxious fascination. The allure of drugs (and their associated evil) renders the unfamiliar familiar, or makes that which is properly kept strange seem like home. Being on drugs means being at home with degradation. Here, the topic of drugs is not an opportunity for thinking about actual material ingestions, but is used to encapsulate the danger of certain social terrains. The thrill of contamination conveyed by watching the well-heeled character Helena forced to walk the same dangerous precinct as the streetwise Mexican policeman Javier in her efforts to maintain her family's affluent lifestyle, or Robert Wakefield surveying (from the safety of his official, anonymized vehicle) the same downtrodden neighborhood that his daughter walks moments later by foot in her quest to score crack, is precisely the currency of the film.[13] The sullying of these vulnerable, hopeful characters is what is at stake—they risk becoming matter out of place. Drugs form a sign of abject displacement in a textual logic that foregrounds the menacing proximity of the socioeconomically and racially dissimilar, the shiftiness of that which is (mis)recognized as home. The sense of unease produced by these referential sequences arouses feelings of estrangement from changing urban cultural topographies, fomenting a misplaced nostalgia for a certain sort of (white) cultural security and centrality.

If the problem the film constructs is Caroline's hazardous inability to distinguish between (or, more accurately, her habit of conflating) home and away, the challenge for her father is to put this confusion straight by finding himself a role most appropriate to the task. This marks out a trajectory from "faceless bureaucrat" (versed in abstract generalities) to "head-of-family man" (with firsthand experience of the problem). Enrolled in the logical momentum of this journey are the many absurdities, failings, and excesses of the war on drugs, as dramatized. The resultant casualties are revealing. When Wakefield first assumes office, he attends an official function along with numerous experts from the drug field. The voices and advice of these experts produce such a cacophony that it's not long before a nonplussed Wakefield is reaching for the scotch. The congenial irony of this scene conveys a subtler intimation: that the lack of a simple, unified stance among the intelligentsia is *productive* of (something like) the problem at hand. The confusion of expert knowledge is further contrasted with the supposed transparency of firsthand experience when a frustrated Wakefield asks an aide to clear his schedule because he's "tired of talking to experts who've never left the beltway. It's time to see the frontlines." The scene switches immediately to one in which Caroline is freebasing in her bathroom in the family home.

Though "on the right track," Wakefield is apparently yet to realize that the "frontlines" of the drug problem *are* the "homes" of America, and in particular *his* home, in which his public commitment has made him a stranger.

Recognizable here are traces of the "culture war" rhetoric used by the former drug czar, William Bennett, who offered himself to the popular imagination as "a liberal who has been mugged by reality."[14] Bennett is well known for characterizing intellectuals, liberal journalists, and, through this filter, anyone who disputes his position on drugs as myopic elites, whose abstract theories blind them to what is plainly apparent to "regular" American people. If, in Bennett's worldview, the university of the late 1960s and "cultural deconstruction" are the environments in which "America lost its moral bearing regarding drugs," *Traffic* takes this association one step further when Caroline and her friends are depicted getting high late one night, unsupervised at an opulent college venue. Amidst their disjointed ramblings (laced with expressions of generational resentment and sexually ambiguous desires), we discern jumbled, half-baked, stuttering objections to "social conventions" and incoherent pledges to "change this whole social pattern." The scene culminates in one friend's violent and convulsive overdose—the lethal, volatile body of the American campus.

The primary narrative culminates with Wakefield quitting office after breaking down giving his maiden speech to the press. Ostensibly the sequence rebukes the rhetoric of the war on drugs. But in its place a sentimental, even more conservative vision of the national future is offered, expressing major disillusionment with the capacities of the state, while consolidating *even more insistently* the criteria of the cultural war that the war on drugs represents:

> The war on drugs is a war that we have to win and a war that we can win. We have to win this war to save our country's most precious resource—our children. Sixty-eight million have been targeted by those perpetrating this war, and protecting these children must be our priority. There has been progress and there has been failure, but where we have fallen short, I see not a problem, I see an opportunity. An opportunity to correct the mistakes of the past while laying the foundation for the future. This takes not only new ideas but per-

severance. This takes not only resources but courage. This takes not only government but families. I've laid out a ten . . . ten point plan that . . . I can't do this. If there is a war on drugs, then many of our family members are the enemy, and I don't know how you wage war on your own family.

At face value, the appeal makes humane sense. But rather than questioning the terms of a system failing people, it makes that system personal. "War" stands in here for all possible embodiments of public action, locking any public future in this area to the failures of the past. In a gesture of atonement, Wakefield abandons the "war" and leaves his office to support his daughter's recovery, embarking on an intimate project— "to listen"—that need only be extended to his immediate kin for him to fulfill his commitment to the nation. The hope extended here is that intimate humane labor (between parents and children) will counterbalance the effects of a market whirling dangerously out of the state's control. This move to retain order in the private realm is meant then as an exemplary attempt to secure a national future unblemished by history or power, where the role of parent comes to exhaust the public dimensions of managing American citizenship.

Race is bound up in this crisis of domestic space in complex ways. In a motif that recurs in this archive the full degradation of drugs is conveyed dramatically when the young female character is forced—through sheer compulsion to sustain her habit—to have sex with a drug dealer, specifically a muscular or otherwise physically domineering African American male drug dealer. In *Traffic* this event takes place downtown in the daytime, to the eerie sounds of children playing outside, and culminates in Caroline beckoning the dealer to inject drugs into her ankle. This "Desdemonic" moment is offered as the ultimate point of danger and depravity, the upraised ankle evoking questions of support and flexibility —a system vulnerable, volatile, stretched to limits. The vision of compulsive femininity in the hands of the racial, economic, and moral other enables *Traffic* to express what it imagines as the incommensurable differences of the worlds through which the drug trade moves and whose extremes it is thought to represent.

It would be a mistake though to interpret *Traffic* in terms of an even logic of exclusion on the basis of race. Its system of value is more brutal and in fact more inclusive. Gilles Deleuze and Félix Guattari offer the concept of faciality as a way of thinking about modern racism that locates its source not in exclusion, but a system of differential inclusion that supposes a basic prepolitical humanity, modeled on "the White-man face."[15] Faciality is a grid that tests humanness according to a logic of personal identification. Patricia MacCormack usefully understands this concept in terms of an inability to recognize the body of the other except as it conforms to the terms of the dominant culture. Faciality thus becomes a refusal to allow the other a viable body at all: "Where the face differs is why the face fails, not because certain genders or races are destined to fail but because certain bodies are wrenched into a facial assemblage destined to fail them."[16] In *Traffic*, transactions with the drug dealer take place through a small caged grid in the latch of a bolted door, through which it is possible to make out a fraction of his face (see figure 2). This threshold is breached only twice in the film, once in the scene described above, and once when Wakefield is searching for his daughter. Both occasions are produced as violent and violating—the release of a dangerous, untamed force. The grid is otherwise in place in the film, grading its characters according to a facial logic that takes its bearings from two complementing axes—involvement in the drug trade and devotion to the national-family form.

Racial difference is tolerated in the world of the film "at given places under given conditions."[17] Jaundiced, bustling streetscapes of poverty are contrasted with the cold, puritanical blue of affluent domesticity (associated with the Wakefields' residence). As effectively as shades of skin, these pigments determine "degrees of deviance in relation to the White-man face."[18] On this coding system, whiteness is less a preexisting attribute than a source of value and aspiration: nonconforming traits are integrated according to its terms, which map only loosely onto racial categories. Ascending from the low points on this ladder of virtue and value are characters like Javier, the Mexican policeman who manages to resist corruption (and precarious offers of family-like loyalty from members of the Juarez cartel) by sticking to his goal of getting lighting installed in Tijuana parks so that children can play baseball at night. ("Everyone likes baseball.")[19] But perhaps the most interesting performance of a sort of cumulative racial-national capital is that of Helena, the unsuspecting wife of a wealthy drug dealer.[20] When she discovers her

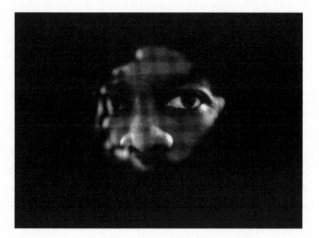

Fig. 2. The dealer's face. Still from *Traffic* (2000).

family's affluent lifestyle and rapid upward mobility have been built on drug crime (her husband is placed in confinement at the start of the film), she is faced with the prospect of a serious reversal of fortune. Catapulted into action when a thug chasing a bad debt threatens to kidnap her son, she takes on aspects of her husband's operation. In so doing, she adopts the conflicted status of a protagonist engaging in the unvirtuous deeds of drug trafficking for purposes nonetheless invested as highly virtuous in the world of the film (protecting her family). This ambiguous relation to the terms of national authority is encapsulated humorously when she takes a tray of lemonade out to a van outside her house in which undercover DEA officers are busy monitoring for any signs of illicit activity. She asks them politely if they could keep an eye out for any signs of danger to her children, constituting herself— momentarily—as a proper beneficiary of, rather than threat to, national protection.

The racial coding of Helena and her family is ambiguous, to say the least. The DEA cops monitoring the case are excited at the prospect of getting "the top people, the rich people, the *white* people!" But Helena distinguishes herself to her friends as "European" at the start of the film; and her darker features (she is played by Catherine Zeta-Jones) and those of her husband, Carlos (played by Steven Bauer), produce some disso-nance on this count. Their character names are marked as exotic, if not distinctly Hispanic. Their surname, Ayala, is distinctly shady. In the logic of faciality, "there are only people who should be like us and whose crime it is not to be."[21] Though devoted to the comfortable family form, these characters are disqualified from whiteness, it would seem, on the basis of their morally suspect involvement in trafficking. They are, in short, not-yet-quite-white.

The drug trade is used to figure Helena's displacement as a strong but palpably vulnerable woman moving in public (albeit criminal), male space. The ambiguous implications of her mission are stressed further by her situation as mother carrying fetus. In Mexico, she reveals to accomplices details of a plan called Project for the Children, an operation in which high-grade cocaine is to be sculpted into the shape of children's toys in order to escape detection at the border. Here Helena is made to *embody* the incompatibility of the domains of parenting and drugs when she risks losing the deal by refusing—on account of being pregnant—to engage in the ritual of testing the drugs that she produces. If Helena's performance as heroic parent shores up her moral status in the film, this status is compromised by the corrupt Project for the Children the film codes as located in the very substance of the traffic in which she trades (kiddies' toys composed insidiously of cocaine). Here her private "mother's instincts" are shown to override the risks of this most repugnant and unauthorized of trades. But these parents' project for their own children is ultimately measured against the generic category of Children that their project is deemed as affecting.

Who are these endangered children? The answer the film gives is Caroline, an "entirely specific" child, which does not preclude her from "acquiring and exercising the most general of functions."[22] Caroline is the uniform image of life that drugs are shown to endanger. Caught using drugs in her bathroom, she swings round to face her father proclaiming "fuck you!" in adult, guttural tones that recall her altogether more abject predecessor, Regan from *The Exorcist* (William Friedkin, dir., 1973). *Traffic*'s overall remedy is not exorcism however, if exorcism is understood as expulsion of the abject other, but rather the implementation of a wavering zone of control, the ferocious intimacy of a precious resource—facetime—that considers all difference amenable to a self-assured uniform standard in order to turn away from a strife-ridden public sphere. So

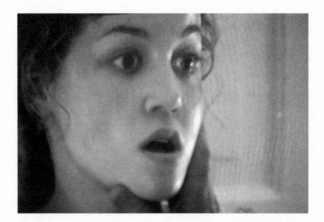

Fig. 3. Caroline confronts her father. Still from *Traffic* (2000).

when Caroline is confronted with her father's authority in this scene, what we end up seeing, as her father cleans out the bathroom, is the volatile labor of incorporation: her face, gaping, stunned, and staggering, propagating "waves of sameness until those who resist identification have been wiped out,"[23] reeling in the process of trying to absorb or reject the multiple divergences from her type encoded, by the film, in the sign of drugs (see figure 3).

Traffic is used to grade families, and families, to guard against traffic in a referential system in which traffic also stands for the perceived dangers and futility of managing a society in which everything is not ultimately the same. The gendered dimensions of this picture become apparent in its complex siting of vulnerability, in which the *child* is exposed, through parental neglect, to the same hazardous excesses of the contemporary world that prevent the *mother* from being able to competently or safely carry out her duty to defend her child.[24] Enter Dad. Within a terrain viewed as teeming with radical, perilous, but aspirationally assimilable differences, a trope of protection is brought into being that conceives racial, economic, and sexual order by confining those marked by these categories to the privileged terms of white nuclear space. Dad's face ciphers and stands in for the face of the nation, the president, the bosom of the White House, all of whose presence is otherwise elusive in the accelerating rush of traffic.

Domesticating Consumption

So far I have examined the availability of the trope of drugs to a privatizing logic of national morality. The protective authoritarianism drugs are thought to call for is easily transplanted from state to family, leaving a rubble of bureaucratic bungling, squandered funds, and undue anguish and violence as evidence for the rightness of this path. But I have also tried to illustrate the fears and desires that animate this narrative—fears of the loss of security and control over the hope of the nation. If Caroline embodies a national character exposed to the control of unfamiliar and alien forces, the story engenders desire for a basic moral alignment that has little time for the historical disparities and economic conditions that produce the misfortunes of the present.

Instead, hopes for social repair are pinned on a fragile and luminous reserve that can be elaborated through the notion of "face-time." *Face-time* connotes access to a pure empathic immediacy and authentic humanity capable of restoring moral order and accommodating difference within a mutually legible system of value. The word *face* evokes a sense of intimacy, suggesting the extracurricular terms of the private sphere. In this compound, *time* implies a fraught relation and potential availability to an economy of labor, indicating a competitive relation with, or subjection to, labor time. *Face-time* must be slotted in, scheduled wherever possible, to do the work of relational maintenance and social repair in a world viewed as increasingly abstract and abstracting. It holds out for a realm of transparent contact and unmediated exchange where the self and its desires are plainly apparent, decipherable, and soluble. In fact, face-time never materializes in the film. Instead, it is suspended tantalizingly, endlessly deferred as a pledge—"to listen"—that represents a disingenuous alternative to the political.

Feminists have highlighted the ambiguous status of women's domestic work and shown how this sort of affective labor is usually relegated to operating *outside* the scope of public transactions, as their necessary but unaccounted prerequisite. But here we have the allocation of this form of intimate labor to the male "head-of-household"—its invocation even in relations between members of public office. Perhaps face-time is not a private matter, after all. Perhaps it connotes face-to-face communication, the paradigm of public discourse and rational-critical dialogue. In fact, *face-time* indicates a merger of these domains in the national imaginary.[25] Now that the dangers, pleasures, and disruptions of the world of exchange are seen to cut across national and traditional borders in ways that apparently escape the state's control, the labor of recognizing and commanding an original, transparent humanity at the base of social transactions assumes increased responsibility—and exercises increased force. In *Traffic*, Barbara Wakefield's provision of mother-to-daughter face-time to Caroline has, by implication, fallen short. Robert Wakefield's assumption of the job only indicates the increased force such a function is expected to exercise when the state is cast as incapable of fulfilling the role of securing order. An authoritative instatement of the national-family form is enlisted to domesticate all exchange and consumption.

But there is an interesting slippage here. Though it is generally *the market* that requires the separation of wage-earners from their dependents, giving rise to circumstances presumed to breed habits such as Caroline's, the offending preoccupation in *Traffic* is identified only, a priori, as "drugs." It is drugs—as a problem of the nation-state—that demand Robert Wakefield's attention and separation from his family. Elided from this picture is the way the organization of labor and demands of capital play into the family's deterioration. Instead, drugs are posed as the conveniently blameworthy substitute. Next, *family* is prescribed as an antidote to the unsatisfactory conditions and unhappy outcomes of deteriorating domestic relations. While drugs are constructed as the primary nuisance to families, only families, in their pure and natural form, can protect against drugs. Families become, in the manner of an infinite regress, both poison and cure—a *pharmakon* of their own—leaving economic conditions uninterrogated.

In this way drugs take on the vague but sweeping symbolic status of that which is felt to be lacking in the present constitution of the nation, acting, in William Connolly's words, as a container for "diffuse feelings of uncertainty, anxiety, and resentment."[26] As Connolly observes, the specific valences of the war on drugs—what it represents and for whom—can change according to cultural variations in the lived experience of insecurity, danger, and displeasure. Among these, he points to the threat of racial violence on the street, the shifting ethnic composition of the population, the loss of work and economic prospects (as projected onto women and minorities thought to have stolen them), the inability of the state to control the effects of economic change, and the rapid pace of cultural shifts in general. Encapsulating the negative affects linked to these concrete experiences of globalization is the particular achievement of the political deployment of drugs. And as a subcategory of the media theme of "law and order," drugs enjoy a further capacity to scare people into increased support for authoritarian measures and styles of government.

This dynamic is entirely pertinent in the Australian context. In her manifesto, *The Truth*, published in 1996, Pauline Hanson, the leader of the One Nation party of Australia, declares that "In our cities, girls as young as 14 sell sex for as little as $10 to buy drugs from Asian gangs."[27] In this image the icon of a compromised will vulnerable to foreign control is as significant as the price of ten dollars. Hanson's subjects weren't just morally imperiled—they were getting *ripped off* in the process. Buoyed by a tide of economic protectionist, anti-immigration, and nationalist-racist sentiment, this extremist party achieved a considerable measure of cultural and political power by stirring economic and cultural disaffection among Anglo- (or "middle") Australians.[28] Yet Hanson was not nearly as successful as her symbolic heir, the former prime minister John Howard, in directing these reactionary sentiments to the purpose of producing a pervasive, suspicious insularity, achieved by floating the ideal of the nuclear family, and thus characterizing domestic space. Howard's discourse managed to inflect the space and time of citizens' ambit of agency in such a way that the familial home came to adopt the symbolic function of the protection people have when they *don't* have economic protectionism. But how did drugs come to figure in this process? And what symbolic mechanisms do they afford?

It may help here to consider the notion of the fetish, psychoanalytically conceived. In this story, the fetish is a defensive mechanism adopted by the male subject to deal with the sight of his penis-less mother. In response to the fear of castration this sight is thought to provoke, the young male libidinally invests in another object, which must operate, ever tenuously, as a substitute phallus. Tenuously, because the subject knows and does not know that the fetish is a mere substitute. The investment flickers tentatively between knowledge and belief, "haunted by the fragility of the mechanisms that sustain it."[29] This story provides one way of conceiving the mutual referentiality of drugs and family (at a social, rather than individual psychosexual level). If drugs operate, as I have argued, to trope a distressing lack in the present tense of globalization, the political fetish they provoke is, by virtue of a well-trodden history of associations, the nuclear family in the home. And, like the fetish, this figure must steep itself in elaborate fictions, contrivances, and massive proportions of wishful energy if it is to adequately fulfill this function. To the liberal imagination, shoring up the safe haven of the home space is an entirely reasonable way of resisting a hazardous, unpredictable, and messy outside. But what is not visible from this perspective is how the family gets invested in this process—as a narrow pedagogical apparatus, an intensified site of responsibility and blame, a pressurized thing that comes to bear more and more of the charge of social harmony in conditions that actively disrupt it.[30]

As though to confirm the existence of these compensatory and circular attachments comes the Australian National Drugs Campaign of 2001. Accompanying the booklet that proposed families as the strongest defense against the drug problem came a series of linked TV ads, which achieved some mention in the critical literature, most notably in Guy Rundle's deft analysis of John Howard's prime-ministership. As Rundle described: "The first part of the campaign featured a couple of grungy scenes—a teenage girl in a dingy room prostituting herself for money to buy drugs, a boy being zipped up into a bodybag. . . . Still more bizarre was the follow-up campaign in which we saw a couple of seconds of the first ad, which then pulled back to reveal a family watching the ad and discussing the dangers of drugs, which pulled back to reveal another family discussing the family discussing the first ad which then . . . and so on in eternal recession."[31] Rundle laughs the first ad off—"pure Fassbinder . . . practically a marketing campaign for the lifestyle"—but I want to take its animation of parental fear more seriously.[32] Piping over its images of everyday despair—teenage prostitution, petty crime, a mother-daughter tussle, and an overdose—come the wavering voices of children telling us what they want to be when they grow up.[33] A mournful register is mustered to depict futures that would have been. The goals are not extravagant: an English teacher, a mother, a fireman, a restaurant owner. But as these modest dreams come into articulation with drugs, a disembodied chorus of personal aspirations offsets and oversees a visual spectacle of disgust, poverty, and despair. It may be stating the obvious to say that this text mimics and organizes a broader sense of cultural nostalgia and loss. Still, its fictive devices remain worth highlighting. These are, after all, not the selfsame voices of the figures depicted visually as degraded or deceased, but retrieved voices speculating what these figures might have become at some point in the future which coincides with (but dramatically offsets) the present envisioned. Though they acquire a disembodied, transcendent quality—hovering somewhere beyond these images—these voices are performing an immanent textual function. They configure a perspective on the present that is continually conditioned by the retrospective, reconstructed hope of a future imagined as lost—as though to conjure a nostalgia for the future.

These are the voices of private aspiration. If Caroline's and Helena's stories in *Traffic* foreground the prominence of the theme of class mobility in contemporary drug narratives, the title of this ad ("Lost Dreams") and contemporaneous texts (the film *Requiem for a Dream*) corroborate it. The loss of dreams, understood as aspirations and ambitions for the future, is the critical motif here. With their intensely personal and intimate tones, the mourned voices prescribe privacy as the safest, most immediate mode of belonging to the future. Drugs are portrayed as a calamitous deviation whose principal effect is to endanger, if not obliterate, the realization of personal hopes and dreams. But what is particularly interesting about this genre is how it exposes and re-exposes the wound at the base of this desire. Drugs materialize as an ever-present possibility of future despair, necessitating prudence. The mobilization in these texts of disgust, which is associated with particular embodiments of taste, and thus of class and class mobility, is also relevant here.[34] If the source of the drug problem, in these stories, is an infirmity lodged deep within the moral fiber of the individual, the dreams that have become impossible as a result, and are thus supposed to have been lost, take on the character of a haunting reminder of what *could have been*, coming to exhaust, with grievous dominance, the conditionality of the present.

The appearance of this theme in drug texts suggests the significance of a sense of endangerment for this conception of the present: the reactive and reactivated underbelly of current notions of "all that's modern, forward-thinking, and entrepreneurial about Australian society."[35] The appearance of the "aspirational voter" served to bolster the claim that policies vouchsafing private provision, rather than redistribution, had most chance of popular support (or at least, the type of popular support that counts). At the time, left commentators were quick to point out that aspiration "is just another word for hope." The Australian journalist Tom Morton wrote that "aspirational politics assumes that our hopes are purely private hopes," aligning a particular set of interests and desires with the national interest, and thereby embodying a very particular "distribution of hope."[36] The drug campaign micromanages this redistribution of hope in its own small way by offering an alternative sense of security than that associated with the welfare state. Markers of national unity take on a heightened significance in this context, as Ghassan Hage argues, because disadvantaged populations must cling to the idea that " 'national identity' is bound to be a passport of hope for them."[37] The last boy in this ad wants to play soccer for Australia, we learn, as his body is zipped up into a body bag. His humbly added "if I'm good enough" cleaves individual determination to moral intent, suggesting it is as much the possession of a national dream, as the plausibility of the dream itself, that qualifies one as a candidate for this expression of national sentiment. One by one, each image is transferred away from the political, materializing as a question of individual determination and moral intent. In a curious funnelling motion, this works to install an insulated view of the future, in which the scope of citizen agency is reduced to narrow proprietary terms.

Whatever disturbances the first ad arouses—the flickers of fear, disgust, grief, nostalgia, and excitement—can take refuge in the slim shreds of hope it offers, a mode of hope that is produced as innocent enough, personal, and constitutively endangered. But if this is not enough, the second ad provides an elaborate model for channeling and domesticating these volatile and unruly fears in a vision of homely security and family togetherness. This second ad performs a didactic function in relation to the first, with an abysmal image of a nation bound only by homes, televisions, and families. Here we are introduced once more to the authoritarian but tender parent, implored to impersonate the state. Her first appearance has her calming her daughter, who is upset watching the initial TV ad (described above) alone in her room. As in *Traffic*, where the privacy of Caroline's bathroom is constructed as a place of suspicion and possible youthful deviance, the placement of the television in the girl's room is rendered ever-so-slightly problematic: a source of disturbance and likely confusion requiring the general guidance a good parent can provide. The parent engages her daughter in a discussion about drugs, and instantaneously, the scene is funneled into television. Now, the parent is the father of an Asian-Australian family, watching this same scene with his two children in their suburban living room. Given the connection in the white Australian psyche between "Asian" gangs and drugs, the family's ethnicity is marked, but here we are presented with the reassuring image of this ever-suspect ethnicity domesticating itself (in a way that *Traffic's* Ayala family never quite succeeds in doing). This expression of ethnicity is contained—suburban, familiar, and homely— not extended, street-based, or altogether strange—and promotes a certain moral identification. The father asks his son about how he would approach an offer of drugs, and suddenly they too are whisked onto TV, suitable viewing for a family of four in a big country house. Our new set of parents' skilled efforts at turning their son's prying questions into an opportunity for instruction are similarly siphoned into the dowdier living room of a family of four, whose respective intent to find out more about the best ways to talk to their children is followed by a brief promotion of the campaign booklet. In the concluding scene, we watch a mother tending to breakfast in a smart kitchen. The camera follows her before stopping to linger on Dad and son, who are starting their day watching the TV promotion for the booklet while eating breakfast at the kitchen table (more about the kitchen table later). As Mum leaves the frame, Dad says, "we should read that," and his son agrees straightforwardly, unhesitatingly.

This extraordinary piece of social marketing activates the postwar construction of the television as a symbol of family "togetherness," so as to convert, in gradual stages, a potentially uncomfortable and awkward mother-daughter situation into a blueprint for straightforward paternal instruction and agreement. The image of families huddled together around television sets bears traces of 1950s discourses, whose suggestion that televisions would bring families closer together (itself a spatial metaphor) contained the conviction that solutions to domestic discord were available through the skillful organization of space.[38] Thus, a scene of teenage exposure and isolation is ameliorated progressively, finally perfected, via a series of corresponding situations, at the morning kitchen table. Contrasting starkly with the harsh, abject scenes of the counterpart ad (a hotel room, a public toilet, a shattered household, and a street at night), the ad also binds itself intimately into the production and allocation of comfortable space. The harsher scenes of the first ad form a constitutive "outside" that works to produce the homely imaginary woven here. We can see here allusions to the "hypodermic model" of media effects, whose concern with mass brainwashing extended to the effects of violence on TV. The disturbing effects of media were supposed to enjoin special efforts on the part of parents to supervise their children's consuming habits. The instruction here for parents to talk to their children about drugs thus becomes a plea for them to domesticate consumption *in general*, with no apparent acknowledgement of the fact that the state has actually *produced* the first ad that it shows parents ameliorating with such exemplarity in the second! The niggling anxiety underscoring the campaign as a whole, then, is that the media does *not*, as this discourse would have it, "reduce everybody to one drugged faceless consumer"[39]—hence the careful enlistment of parents in the second ad to that purpose! And while it may be that, if presumed effective, this crude attempt at social engineering belies at least some degree of confidence in the "hypodermic model" of reception it admonishes, the effectivity of the campaign does not lie so much in the way it manages to dupe its consumers. Rather, it lies in its aptitude for touching and arousing tangible fears—of family breakup or tragedy, crime, theft, attack, or loss of property—"and since it promulgates no other remedies for their underlying causes, it welds people to that 'need for authority' which has been so significant for the right in the construction of consent to its authoritarian programme."[40]

Such authority is situated as securable with and within the family—in particular, the masculine embodiment of home command. But family is also, in this appellation, a highly leveraged product. Guy Rundle is quick to observe the emphasis here on "training families to behave as families, as if they could no longer be trusted to perform that duty without prompting."[41] He continues, "The idealized social relationship between the family and the state was thus reversed: instead of the family being the ground of society upon which the state and law rested, the family was reconstructed as an arm of the state, to whom was subcontracted the role of shaping the behaviour of the young, in a manner scripted by professionals."[42] As many have argued, the dream of strengthening traditional social forms does not involve the retrieval of an actually forsaken past, but demands the production of ever *new* forms, importuned to contend with the present social order. Here, the parent attains the status of "the new virtuous category of majority."[43] Meanwhile, the uniform arrangement of national-domestic space (figured to consist entirely of families around televisions in homes, drawn together against a hostile and threatening outside) directs attention toward subtle gradations of affluence and respectability among them, enabling a practice of incremental comparison to take place. Relations based on alternate bonds—ethnicity, sexuality, class, friendship—are disregarded in favor of an axis of familiar-national aspiration. A grid of nuclear homes conjoined by mass media is what it must take to make the nation a home in this vision of domesticating consumption.

Before proceeding, it is worth contemplating how this coding of domestic space played out in the political unconscious of the Australian federal election in 2001. The appearance of a $27.5 million initiative as part of the Liberal party's re-election campaign "to develop and introduce retractable needles and syringes to protect the public from needle-stick injury leading to HIV infection" was perhaps the most topical of its material ramifications: "Many parents of young children, whose great fear when their children are out playing in the park or on the beach are [*sic*] needles, will welcome this initiative very warmly," Howard was quoted as saying, without noting the complete absence to date of any reported instances of infection in Australia by these means.[44] Parents and their charges were taken to coincide with "the public" at the expense of other, more pertinent subjects. But there were further, more oblique traces of this broad shift in the national-cultural constitution at this time. While opposition leader Kim Beazley made a point of campaigning steadfastly on "domestic" issues—health, jobs, and education—Howard had already characterized domestic space in terms conducive to his cultural program, leaving the opposition to play hopelessly to his cultural specifications. Amplified by the threats thought to be posed to national security by the *Tampa* affair and September 11, the election saw Howard campaigning on "certainty, leadership, and strength," a situation that involved a bizarre gendering of the electorate, in which the perceived "strength" of the candidates was endlessly calculated, Howard touted as "Iron Johnny" and the "Ladies' Man"—"Women will see Howard home."[45] If the *Tampa* case was, as some commentators observed, experienced by many as a law-and-order issue (court cases involving gang rapes by men of "Middle Eastern background" dominated tabloid newspapers and talkback radio well before the *Tampa* incident), it also illustrated the changed terms of national racism. While racial prejudice undoubtedly colored popular attitudes to the asylum seekers, it is significant that race itself was not the basis of exclusionary rhetoric. Rather, the asylum seekers' deficit of national belonging was publicized in the highly fabricated terms of their moral status as *parents*. Photographs suggesting that children had been thrown overboard were used by the government to propagate the view that the asylum seekers were unsuitable—too inhuman, in fact—to become part of the Australian community. This ground of exclusion carried all the more significance given that the category of "economic refugee" (the "non-genuine" asylum seeker) might otherwise be considered the aspirational subject par excellence.

After a desperate last-minute dash on the eve of the election on Beazley's part to get through to "the kitchen table of the average Australian family," "where ordinary Australians are doing it tough," newspapers announced Howard's victory by proclaiming, "Suburbs make a fellow feel at home"—a motif anticipated some weeks earlier in Paul Kelly's "When Johnny Comes Marching Home."[46] In the aftermath of the election, Beazley was left to ponder the key to re-establishing social unity, which, he proposed—in remarkably acquiescent imagery—was to look "to security in the hearts and minds of those around the kitchen table." He proclaimed, "We have looked down through the fog of war to the kitchen table of the average Australian family . . . We've listened to their hopes and their dreams."[47] My suggestion is that this kitchen table is the very same piece of national-symbolic furniture assigned the task of resolving, through deferral, our *mise en abyme* of drugs, families, homes, and televisions. As a scene of national aspiration and civil correspondence, it "neutralizes in advance any expressions or connections unamenable to the appropriate significations."[48] Its mood of homely readiness and seemingly natural demarcation of gender roles, its no-nonsense configuration of paternal dictation and parental guidance, its appeal to the "middle Australia" it actually functions to constitute, and its transcendence of other forms of social affiliation—these aspects combine to provide an exemplar of domesticated consumption and civil coincidence in the Australian present tense, one that is continually reproduced and naturalized by drugs and other fear-inducing tropes on "outside" space. But this iconic scene of national action and affiliation does a great disservice to the "ordinary Australians" it tries to woo, not only by foreclosing and depreciating other forms of social and political relation or by transmitting a collective temperament of suspicious insularity, but also because of the complacency inherent in its tendency to refer the challenges of globalization back onto this fetishized and overinvested form. Just as feminist critics of psychoanalysis advise against confusing the penis with the phallus, it is worth recalling at this point that drugs do not equal the social dangers that political and economic injustices engender—nor "the family" a sole, fair, or sufficient way of coping with them.[49] In short, these media not only dramatize, but also serve to *compound* the disastrous frustration of dreams of a better life that do not accord with a privatized future of white middle-class heterosexuality.

Aspiration Dependency

Critics and commentators from the left have become fond of identifying sexual politics with market forces. In this view, the sexual revolution destroyed the family; thus feminists and others appear as willing accomplices in a consumerist agenda that whittles away any remaining defenses against global capital, the family appearing as the last unit separating the individual from the market, the last bastion of human intimacy and community.[50] As I have argued, the consumer context has certainly shaped the politics of identity in specific ways. But this left-conservative attitude profoundly mistakes the shape of contemporary power. In particular, it misses the ways in which the family itself has become subject to a politico-cultural commodity fetish. You will recall from the last chapter how, from the Frankfurt School perspective, the commodity is invested with the hope of overcoming the alienated condition, only to wrench human relations further apart and condemn the consumer to a perpetual "re-creation of frustration." This dynamic is figured most potently in these images of domesticated consumption, where it appears, almost despite itself, as an endlessly self-referential recursive or addictive structure.

This insight informs the narrative of the film *Requiem for a Dream*

(Darren Aronofsky, dir., 2000), in which Sara, a lonely widow, gets wrapped up in the idea of being on television when she receives a canvassing call from her favorite game show. In a moment of excitement and nostalgia, she vows to wear the red dress she wore to her son Harry's graduation: a relic of family togetherness and pride. But she finds she's too big to fit into the red dress. She begins a cycle of dieting and soon finds herself embroiled in a vexing battle of wills with her refrigerator. With her doctor's prescription, she enlists the help of diet pills, which thrillingly propel her one small step along her arc of self-realization. But the game show doesn't call again, and soon the pills stop delivering the same giddy sense of momentum and accomplishment. With her hopes pinned on a call from the show, her feelings of remorse and loneliness grow. The longer her dream fails to materialize, the more her obsession to manifest this token of past togetherness intensifies. In desperation, she ups the dose of her diet pills, and on the story speeds—to its harrowing and horrific conclusion.

One of the agonizing features of this narrative is the individualizing force of Sara's desire. Though initially she involves others in her project, she neglects and eventually rejects the company of a large group of friends on her block (other elderly widows) as a source of possibility and satisfaction, declaring, simply, "It's not the same!" The focal effect of her desire (to lose weight to fit into the red dress to be on the game show to recuperate an earlier moment of happiness and togetherness) pulls her further and further away from any exploration or enjoyment of these proximate and potential relations.[51] It is as though the image of the dream becomes so consuming that it obliterates any real chance of approximating the happiness it so rigidly represents. Instead it comes to assume the character of a haunting reminder of what could have been, magnifying the isolation of her present situation and acquiring a disastrous and amplifying momentum of its own.

The television works again in this film as a glorified symbol of family togetherness. But *Requiem* manages to stage this glorification, revealing its character as a fetishized referent for a form of hope that is vigorously deferred. The abysmal nature of this bind appears in miniature in the opening credits, where Harry, Sara's son, is shown trying to convince his mother to unlock the TV, which is secured against thieves, or so she claims. Next, Harry and a friend are shown dragging the television across a desolated landscape of pure recreation—Coney Island—before pawning it for money to buy drugs. Later, Sara is pictured buying the TV back from the pawn shop; a regular occurrence, we are given to believe. Set in an economy that depends for its continuance upon the radiation and atomization of insatiable desires, it is as though the moment Sara places her faith in the family as a haven of trust and security (by unlocking the television), she is forced to meet the costs of her naïve but indispensable belief, something she is prepared and even eager to do, if only to take refuge in its simulated and ever-receding promise of satisfaction and comfort.

In their analysis of urban change in Western Sydney, the urban geographers Brendan Gleeson and Bill Randolph track the purported "movement of young families and retired people from troubled neighbourhoods to the relative stability of the urban fringe"—the sort of movement that the term *aspirational society* attempts to capture.[52] As they explain, the progressive erosion of public resources in the West (transport, hospitals, schools) has raised the appeal of various forms of escape. For some, this entails investment (often under considerable financial pressure) in the "pleasures of order, homogeneity, and amenity" that appear to be offered by the "security communities" located on the urban fringe.[53] For others, it involves various forms of escape and profit represented by the market in drugs and other illicit commodities. Drugs and crime certainly top the list of popular concerns in this region. They seem to encapsulate the experience and apprehension of a progressively degraded public landscape. But, as Gleeson and Randolph demonstrate, the idealized enclaves of family and home that appear to "the more affluent and the more anxious" as viable alternatives to this landscape do not represent a progressive relinquishing of dependence on the state, as many assume. "Far from being simple testimonies to the rewards for individual effort and thrift, these 'landscapes of self-reliance' are in fact heavily dependent upon public subsidies and public endeavour for their creation and maintenance."[54] They are the outcome, that is, of public subsidization of private ways of life (in the form of state subsidization of first-home ownership, and various other private schemes and tax cuts). The term the authors coin for this phenomenon is *aspiration dependency*. "From a societal perspective, aspiration dependency is an expensive habit that is difficult to break by political means. Once hooked on subsidies, affluent

households are not likely to support policies that support a more egali-
tarian and sustainable distribution of social resources and life opportunities."[55] The vocabulary of drugs spontaneously reappears. *Requiem for
a Dream* maps this geography of addiction in psychic terms. In a halluci-
natory and terrifying development, the characters and machinery of the
game show Sara idolizes suddenly burst out of the TV and force their way
into her living room. As well as throwing the poverty of her actual
circumstances into sharp and taunting relief, this exposes in lurid detail
the paraphernalia and multiple intrusive contraptions it takes to sustain
the fetishistic illusion of her desire. The elaborate mechanisms sustaining the romantic investment in "family" intrude here with such force
and volume that Sara is driven—plainly mad—out of her home. *Requiem
for a Dream* identifies the addictive structure of attempts to secure a
future that is framed nostalgically and idealistically as entirely continuous with the past. It provides a critique of the tragic effects of an ever-
narrowing political economy of hope. Given the overbearing moral tem-
plate of addiction that the narrative adopts, the most common response
to the film is a feeling of despair. But the film can also be read as a
prompt to take hold of the queer innovations and combinations that are
actually embodied in the present.

5

CONSUMING COMPLIANCE

. . .

Remembering Bodies Inhabit
Pharmaceutical Narratives

"One influential interpretation of queer studies' appearance in the United States," writes Susan Stryker,

> is that the AIDS crisis necessitated a profound rethinking of the rela-
> tionship between sexuality, identity and the public sphere. Countering
> the homophobic characterization of AIDS as a "gay disease" required
> a postidentity sexual politics that simultaneously acknowledged the
> specificity of various bodies and sexualities (such as gay men) while
> also fostering strategic political alliances between other, sometimes
> overlapping constituencies similarly affected by the epidemic (ini-
> tially African refugees in Europe, Haitians in the United States, hemo-
> philiacs, and injection drug users). This new "queer" politics, based on
> an array of oppositions to "heteronormative" social oppression rather
> than a set of protections for specific kinds of minorities that were
> vulnerable to discrimination, radically transformed the homosexual
> rights movement in Europe and America.[1]

Stryker discusses how the political and intellectual ferment of queer theory enabled transgender activists to formulate "compelling claims that they, too, had political grievances against an oppressive hetero-normative regime." Similarly, this book could be considered continuous with, or closely allied with, this expansive critical project. In tracing how new forms of normativity coalesce around categorizations of drug use, and in considering how these forms of normalization implicate matters of sexuality, gender, class, and race, I hope to have generated further bases for forging political connections and alliances across these

issues that might stand to counter the forms of containment, sectoraliza-
tion, and identity politics that so often characterize the field of public
health. In approaching neoliberal drug discourse as a field of normativity
that regulates and enforces so-called "healthy" consumption, I have
shown how relations of corporeality, subjectivity, temporality, and consumption take shape within a broader field of bionormalization that
distributes hope and life chances unevenly. At the same time I have
attempted to map some of the political technologies, modes of subjectivity, and somatic experience through which these forms of regulation
take hold. I have argued that neoliberal drug discourses are deployed
ideologically to produce a privatization of consumption, engendering a
fearful relation to the future and to others, and producing effects that
are paradoxically analogous to "addiction." By approaching drug discourses as exemplary of a wider field of bionormalization, I have tried
to give a sense of how bionormalization reduces the possibilities (and
indeed the safety) of consumers in a wide range of social locations. A
queer historical approach seeks to provide conceptual resources that
might inform various struggles that are usually considered discrete and
generate some basis for the formation of new alliances, links, and cross-
fertilizations among differently situated struggles, in which questions of
social noncompliance and the consumption of medicine are pertinent.
This does not diminish the need, however, for specific analyses of specifically situated bodies—as Stryker perceptively acknowledges above. Corporeal practice takes shape culturally and contextually, and modes of
resistance to the totalizing procedures of drug discourse (among other
forms of bionormalization) emerge differently from different social locations, almost by definition. It is impossible to elaborate practical forms
of resistance to these normalizing procedures without reference to certain embodied specificities—though identifying the contours of prevailing forms of totalization may well open up unexpected connections
between different struggles that become mutual sources of learning and
transformation.

In the remainder of the book, I consider some of the ways in which
embodied subjects in Western gay locations have resisted and reworked
the discourse of compliance in the interests of well-being. If drug discourses tend to insist that safety and responsibility consist in the individual's rational compliance with the social authority of medicine, gay men's

HIV education has relied effectively on a different set of practices entirely, where safety has depended, not simply on individual compliance with the rational authority of medicine, but on careful experimentation and embodied improvisation on the part of the subjects of medical discourse. In order to understand the field of gay men's responses to HIV/AIDS, I draw on certain insights from corporeal feminism, which, among its other contributions, has developed a different perspective on the possibilities of agency and responsibility than that which is prescribed within medico-moral regimes.[2] In particular, corporeal feminism has developed a notion of ethical agency that is grounded in specific habits of embodiment and practices of inhabitation.[3] This concept of ethics contrasts with conventional understandings that cast ethics as a universal set of principles that are grasped and applied by the rational mind in a disciplinary feat of mind over matter. From the corporeal perspective, ethics are grounded in specific practices of embodiment that are historically conditioned. Ethics involve taking up a position in relation to others, and the sorts of positions it becomes possible to take are laid down in the body through habituation and history. In this sense, responsiveness to a given situation, and to others, is not a function of a mind abstracted from worldly relations applying universal rules straightforwardly to homogenous bodies, space, or practice. Rather, it is enacted through the body, in relation, and through the activation of certain capacities that have been given through one's socially acquired disposition and historically shaped sensibilities. From this perspective, embodied capacities are intricately entwined with social location and historically formed. To understand what a body is capable of, one must understand these processes of historical and social enculturation, and work with the historical resources a given body has at its disposal. In short, it makes no sense to enter into a discussion of agency, responsibility, responsiveness, or resistance, without also considering the historical and social specificity through which particular capacities, attributes, and possibilities are embodied. Medical subjects are also remembering bodies, and they inhabit narratives of compliance and consumption in specific, and specifically resistant, ways.

This approach to embodied ethics and sensibilities is intended to illustrate the possibilities of a broader approach to health responsiveness that attends to specific cultural or embodied repertoires, thus challenging the premium placed on the compliant and abstract or individualized consumer of medicine within psycho-medical discourse. This chapter focuses in particular on gay and HIV-positive responses to HIV antiretroviral therapy, which was made more widely available in Western countries in effective combinations in 1996. Though by no means homogeneous, gay men could be considered to share a specific social positioning which is not entirely undone by the fact that this positioning is differently experienced according to social gradients of race, class, and gender comportment, and which has relatively distinct, if loosely assembled and constantly reassembled, cultural attributes and features. Historically, the response of this group to the threat of HIV/AIDS has activated certain characteristic attributes and dispositions found within its culture, in individual and collective moves that have contested and reworked social and medical prescriptions significantly. Relevant to the approach to embodied agency that this reading develops is the literature on active consumption, which may be adapted to bring the embodied and collective dimensions of the activity of consumption into focus. Health responses do not simply work by prioritizing the rational consumption of medical artifacts. They involve embodied experimentation and collective improvisation on the part of affected groups—forms of labor that may be more or less recognized or denied within given sociopolitical conditions. By focusing on culturally given modes of consumption, I draw attention to the embodied work of specifically located consumers, their reworking of the categories of "health," and some of the specific cultural repertoires, collective dispositions, and processes of enactment by means of which "health" has not simply been consumed, but more viably *produced*. If the discourse of compliance involves a peremptory repudiation of pleasure consuming medicine, a focus on practices of cultural consumption may provide a more capacious perspective on the possibilities of pleasure.

In the previous chapter we were left with the nightmarish image of an isolated widow obsessing to the point of psychosis over a nostalgic ideal of family togetherness and personal fortune propagated by a mass-mediated game show. This chapter opens with another game show, not televised but live, which has traveled around Australia playing mostly to people with HIV (mainly pensioners on low incomes or living in poverty):[4]

The game show revolves around a Chocolate Wheel. Affixed to the wheel are the names of antiviral side effects—neuropathy, say, or insomnia—as well as organs commonly affected by these effects (like the liver). The wheel also includes other aspects of life where HIV drugs might have an effect, such as libido. A member of the audience is called up to spin the wheel. Where the wheel stops, the pointer will indicate that side effect.

Vanessa Wagner then asks the participant about that side effect, using multiple choice answers. The person is presented with a prize regardless of whether their answer is right or not. Prizes are donated by supportive local businesses. Vanessa, Nurse Nancy and an assembled panel of four experts from the HIV sector discuss the particular side effect . . . When the discussion has run its course, the next competitor is called up. And round it goes.[5]

Hosted by drag performer and political activist Vanessa Wagner (Tobin Saunders) and sexpert comedienne Nurse Nancy (Kath Albury), the *Wheel of Misfortune* explores some of the practical challenges of living with HIV treatments in a format that purports not to adhere strictly to a formal "health promotion" model but describes itself rather as "edutainment."[6] The model here, of course, is *Wheel of Fortune*, a game show that pitches itself to "middle Australia" with blatantly "aspirational" content. The *Wheel of* Mis*fortune* uses camp comedic styles to deflate the promises of commercialized medicine and bring them back down to earth, where real people take treatments and live with their unpredictable and frequently messy effects. This is an example of what I describe as "counterpublic health"—the cultivation of viable ethics and modes of embodiment that contend not only with the challenges of HIV infection, but also the mass mediation and medico-moralization of pleasure and health. The *Wheel of Misfortune* achieves this by juxtaposing the commercial game show of self-realization against the lived experience of Highly Active Antiretroviral Therapy (HAART), making a sort of counterpublic out of bodies on treatment.[7] To register the value of this intervention, we need to give up, for a moment, the overbearing standards of evidence propounded by the randomized controlled trial and turn instead to questions of history and cultural value, to embodied and engaged practices of interpretation and response.

The Undetectable Crisis

The highly publicized effectiveness of protease inhibitors and combination therapy at the International AIDS Conference in 1996 ("the Vancouver conference") heralded profound changes in the apprehension of AIDS in the West.[8] I use the term *apprehension* here in both its senses—as perception and as anticipation marked by anxiety or fear. It's a useful term, because it alludes to how perception implies some embodied orientation or affective response. And for many prevention specialists, the new treatments raised, precisely, a deficit of apprehension. Increases in unsafe sex were conceived either in purely rational terms—in terms of a "mistaken belief" that new treatments were a cure—or else in terms of misleading experience, the decreasing signs of the crisis having created a troublesome decline in fear. This led to several arguably disingenuous forms of education, which either insisted in factual terms that the threat of AIDS remained unchanged or else sent researchers scurrying to quantify whether fear was an effective motivator. The logic here was that if the threat of AIDS had declined in visibility, the task for educators was to provide a sort of fear-supplementation—the idea being to keep the fear "real."

Eric Rofes provided a comprehensive and unabashedly personal account of the post-Vancouver period in gay urban centers, which he nicknamed the "Protease Moment." This expression encapsulates well the interlocking processes of medical and consumer fetishism at work "when all social and cultural changes in our experiences of the AIDS epidemic were explained in light of the new therapies."[9] Rofes contests this interpretation by insisting there were changes to gay men's sexual cultures that occurred independently of protease inhibitors. While I think this is true and share many of Rofes's concerns, I wonder if the desire to keep things completely separate doesn't reproduce the notion of the social and the biomedical as independent and discrete spheres—as though the social were not affected by the products of capitalized medicine and as though these products were not the outcome of specific social practices and frames of reference. I believe we need an account of this moment that situates it in terms of a broader politics of knowledge and consumption—a politics that cuts across commercial and socio-sexual domains.

The Protease Moment can be understood in terms of two correspond-ing developments that newly articulated HIV subjects at this time: a luminous material culture generated by the marketing practices of phar-maceutical companies and a discourse of patient compliance associated with the new treatments. The pivotal development of the Vancouver conference was not so much the announcement of a new class of drugs (protease inhibitors), but the ascendancy of a new clinical test, the viral load test, which set new standards for clinical activity and conscious-ness.[10] The viral load test measured rates of viral replication in plasma—an "undetectable" result indicating a rate of viral replication below the test's levels of detection. Recorded on a logarithmic scale, the ability of the viral load test to depict apparently teeming levels of viral activity in the bodies of even asymptomatic patients challenged the notion of a latent period of HIV infection, suggested by the method of monitoring immune function in immunology. What science now "knew" about HIV was that there was no dormant period of infection: the body could now be envisaged as fighting a continuous battle against the virulent activity of HIV. Data were presented indicating that viral load was the best predictor of death and immune decline, while other studies showed that treatment combinations involving a new class of drugs, protease inhibi-tors, were capable of keeping levels of the virus below the test's level of detection. These two findings converged to produce radical new man-dates for therapy. An undetectable viral load became the new standard of clinical practice and patient aspiration. The ability of the new test to quantify an identifiable enemy was met with an equally evocative clinical imperative that emerged as though incontestable from this epistemologi-cal groundswell: Hit Hard, Hit Early.

It is difficult to convey the levels of personal, political, and emotional energy that were directed toward this new objective. In the *Sydney Star Observer*, one gay community activist chided people who refused to accept therapy as "stupid" and a "let down" to the community.[11] In a local HIV-positive publication, one letter writer who voiced his refusal of early intervention on the basis that he had never been sick was pilloried as "delusional" and "under a very serious misapprehension" by another: "The truth is that the virus is replicating voraciously and, as a direct consequence, is placing an enormous burden on his body's immune system."[12] Not all clinicians were as convinced of the practical implications of the truth of viral load testing, pointing to the lack of clinical trials that documented the effects of the drugs over the long term and the complete absence of any long-term data on the effectiveness of early intervention as a strategy.[13] The test was only one of a number of frames, which offered, at best, only a *partial* perspective on the condition of HIV bodies. But for many at this time, the viral load test became the central optic through which the truth of HIV was to be determined, trumping other measures of HIV health.

Out of this epistemological shift emerged a new culture of health imperatives for people living with HIV and, thus, new ontologies of HIV disease. Antiretroviral drugs gained new significance in the treatment imagination. To give some idea of this, where in January 1996 less than 15 percent of HIV-positive gay men surveyed in Sydney were using anti-retroviral therapies, by December 1997 this figure had grown to over 60 percent.[14] Also, before 1997 the uptake of such treatments bore strong associations with declining health, evidenced in HIV-related illness. However, after that time, many more people began taking antiretroviral treatment when feeling well. Previously a strategy adopted in the context of declining health or a reaction to HIV clinical symptoms, treatment now represented a more general endeavor to maintain health. But health had acquired persuasive new terms of reference. The aim of therapy was viral suppression, ideally to keep the level of virus in the blood at "un-detectable" levels. A favorite way of explaining this likened HIV-disease to a train speeding toward a broken bridge. The viral load was the speed of the train; the CD4 (immune function) count was the distance from the site of doom.[15] Health became the carefully managed operation of "stopping the train." This task was complicated by the nature of combination treatment regimes, which were found to require a very high level of regimen compliance to allay the development of viral resistance and to keep the virus at undetectable levels. Michael Flynn registered the initial shock of this new regime of self-management: "We have all had to re-arrange our daily living schedules to fit the drugs in at the right time and dosage. Our whole life is now regimented by our intake of anti-viral drugs. Going out to dinner, meeting friends for a drink, staying away from home or partying all night long have now to be carefully planned like a military operation."[16] The question of when to start ther-apy was typically framed in quasi-devout terms: according to one popular view people were not ready to start until they had "thought and talked it through and [were] ready to make the commitment to stick with it religiously."[17] What was significant about this new regime of self-management was not just the onerous bodily burden that treatment compliance involved—the demanding nature of pill regimes that initially involved dosing two or three times a day, with at least three different classes of drugs, at strict time intervals and sometimes modification of diet—but also its shaping of new HIV subjectivities and bodies.[18] The therapeutic goal of viral suppression oriented the HIV-positive subject in new ways toward the future. The imperative to remain "undetectable" produced the always-present possibility of detecting HIV, inducing a process of constant monitoring and vigilance around the presence of the virus at the level of the individual. Health became an object of very precise, calibrated, forward-looking management—in terms that bore little reference to bodily experience in the world. That is to say, the drugs produced bodies that frequently exceeded common conceptions of health. The ability to endure a range of enervating physical and emotional drug effects was constructed as the natural propensity of moral, self-disciplined subjects.[19] For those who had access to the new treatments and tests, HIV now became visible as a private responsibility, as a "chronic manageable illness," as something about which it would be shameful to make too much of a fuss.

The privatization of the experience of HIV was valued in various ways by people with HIV and was not straightforwardly a negative trend. The suppression of the virus was experienced by many as an opportunity to return to a "normal" life. For those who enjoyed access, treatments generally increased immune function and reduced the risk of dying within ten years of contracting HIV.[20] But for many, viral management presented as an onerous task, the medication viewed as a constant reminder of HIV status. The prospect of "re-engagement" also challenged some aspects of identity developed in response to HIV status, posing difficulties in terms of facing an unexpected future and presenting complex questions about returning to work and reshaping relationships.[21] In its most difficult articulation, a sense of isolation characterized some HIV-positive experience. This was exacerbated by the perseverance of a range of amorphous physical and emotional conditions—"low-level chronic ickiness," as the AIDS educator Ross Duffin has described it.[22]

The changed terms of HIV subjectification played out in tensions that emerged in the People Living with HIV/AIDS (PLWHA) movement in Australia. In a curious way, the introduction of HAART revealed, as though for the first time, the disparities in HIV experience. Now in fact PLWHA had always come from all walks of life—there had *always been* disparity in experience. But where previously people with HIV shared with relative unanimity the sense of a future they wished to avoid and built practices and relations based on this shared aspiration, now the practice of avoiding an unwanted future seemed to have collapsed into personal acts of consumption and compliance, which bore no virtual or necessary relation to others. There appeared to be no shared basis for politics, and the movement was hounded by claims of its failure to represent each and every member. The PLWHA movement had always borrowed heavily from the terms of identity politics to sustain a sense of popular participation and representation, and this encouraged a belief that the expression and representation of embodied particularity was the goal of political aspiration. In the presence of HAART, embodied experience had become fractured along entirely new lines, with some enjoying the benefits from therapy and with others experiencing substantial difficulties and poor clinical results. But this explanation is not adequate in itself to account for the dissension that occurred at this time: after all, there had always been disparate experiences of illness and health among PLWHA, yet the sense of a common predicament had endured. What had changed was not the extent of diversity of positive experience, but *the sort of work* that people were encouraged to perform upon themselves in their avoidance of HIV.[23] The space of the future had been reconfigured, to be filled with aspirations that, under the logic of identity, were supposed to emanate from some interior essence or self. But for some, this self had actually been forged from the social and cultural practices of fighting AIDS, so the apparent determination of this objective by medical science made their lives seem empty or meaningless. This manifested in some accounts in terms of a strange sense of hollowness: "So now, as the epidemic whimpers past its twentieth birthday, we find ourselves in an odd halfway house between death and life, despair and freedom. There is no cure but few people in Australia are actually dying. . . . We are no longer living with death all around us, but we cannot consign the dead to the past and deal with our grief and fear. All we can do is try to forget as much as we can and get on with the rest of our lives, creating for ourselves not a normal existence but an analogue of normality."[24]

Rather than becoming invisible, then, HIV became visible in different ways, through different techniques, and in different concentrations and intensities. The epidemic now appeared as an aggregate of disparate individuals with viruses capable of being managed by these individuals, "in partnership" with doctors. This characterization of the epidemic extended with new force also to the context of HIV prevention, which saw increased use around the world of criminal provisions to prosecute individuals for passing on the virus and increased calls for mandatory testing, name reporting, and partner notification. What had previously been viewed, to a greater or lesser extent, as a shared risk and a shared responsibility—necessitating a range of "shared" practices (such as condom use, volunteerism, and care practices)—was now naturalized as the special responsibility of HIV-positive individuals: "The solution needs to come from within the community, and especially from within the community of HIV-infected people. It is up to us, the HIV-infected, to take charge of this issue *as we have taken charge of our disease*, and let the infection stop with us" (emphasis added).[25]

If AIDS had previously been a very public crisis, enjoining the appropriation of public, social space—evidenced in events such as the AIDS quilt, the Candlelight Rally, the very public activism of ACT UP—the second half of the 1990s saw a withdrawal into the realm of the private. But in constructing this narrative, we are put in the morbid position of romanticizing mass gay death as some sort of precondition to genuine sociality and political transformation. This is precisely the bind in which many people whose lives had been affected by the epidemic now found themselves—their aspirations lurching unsatisfactorily between a frustrating politics of identity, a nostalgic politics of community, or else bland acquiescence to an overtly commercialized normality. What is curious is that the post-Vancouver rush of antiviral enthusiasm traded in remarkably similar terms. One illustration of this comes in the form of an advertisement for Vertex Pharmaceuticals. The AIDS quilt is depicted through a grainy red lens, a thing of the past. Against this background is emblazoned the slogan "Ambition Will Cure AIDS Before Compassion Does" (see figure 4). The ad displaces the collective politics of AIDS organizing with a message of capitalist ambition and entrepreneurial

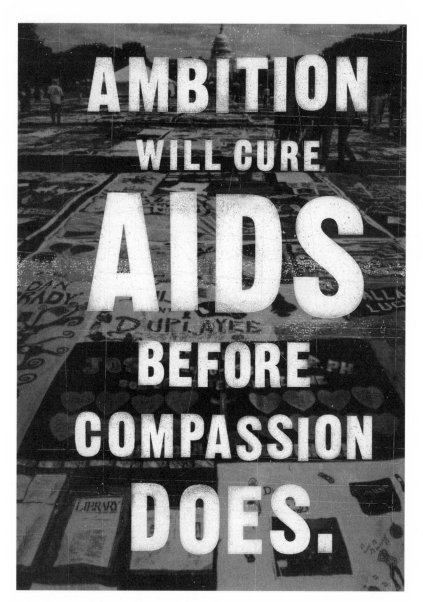

Fig. 4. Vertex Pharmaceuticals advertisement

value. But what is especially interesting is that the social is not quite erased here. It is right there, in fact, larger than life, providing the nostalgic backdrop against which current advances are promoted. The characters of the text are rough-hewn, as though fresh from the pamphlet press of activists. There is a certain sentimental hankering here for the days of crisis, when politics were authentic and community pure. A break is staged between individual rational progress ("ambition") and an equally individual moral quality ("compassion"), which is coded as out-of-date—though not without a tinge of nostalgia. I am reminded here of the politics of aspiration, which pretends "our hopes are purely private hopes."[26] It's easy to read this as a choice between two alternative sets of personal values—one modern, one traditional—when surely both values are compatible, shared, and available to be carried together into the future.

The Vertex ad targets the quandary I have described in HIV political subjectification. It was only one of many drug advertisements that flooded the visual space of HIV in North America, hastened by the relaxation of the U.S. Food and Drug Administration's restrictions on direct-to-consumer advertising. These ads created heated debate about the visual representation of HIV, but the political question hinged less upon the progressive representation of people living with HIV/AIDS than the propensity of these high-gloss ads to encourage unsafe sex. The ads, which typically depicted young people engaged in activities like biking or mountain climbing, seemed to present a problem to the precise extent that they made living with HIV seem possible and occasionally even pleasurable—one San Francisco epidemiologist going so far as to accuse drug companies of "using sex to sell drugs."[27] What was less often acknowledged was the crisis in health promotion the ads had precipitated and how this was framing people's perspectives. The historic reliance on social marketing and its deployment of advertising genres as a principal means of conducting prevention education meant the ads could not avoid being apprehended through particular professional frames. From the idea that safe sex advertisements could suffice as prevention education and sustain safe behavior, it seemed quite plausible that these other advertisements might be largely responsible for destroying it. San Francisco's Stop AIDS Project even attempted to counter this glossy visual landscape by making a spectacle of the disfiguring and less pleasant aspects of HIV treatment, stigmatizing sweating, wasting, bloated, and shitting PLWHA on large billboards in their "HIV is no picnic" campaign.

Less audible in these debates was consideration of how the mediation of HIV-positive lives had become hostage in new ways to broader imperatives—whether those of prevention education or pharmaceutical marketing. While critics of the ads often couched their pleas in terms of "more realistic" representations of living with HIV, the question of *what sort of* reality had become massively overdetermined. The activist Jeff Getty staked out his prescription bluntly: "We don't think it's a sexy disease. It's not about climbing mountains. It's about IV poles, wheelchairs and pain."[28] Little wonder that the pleasure depicted in drug company advertisements held a more hopeful status for some. As Michael Hurley pointed out, "For all the associated problems, drug company advertisements are as likely, if not more likely, to image having a life as a positive person than are the social media."[29] In Australia, where exposure to the ads was limited to imported magazines and internet media, a slightly different take on the protease representational landscape developed. One of the most insightful perspectives came from HIV educator Alan Brotherton, who outlined some of the forces constraining HIV-positive representations:

> Mentioning HIV and pleasure in the same breath is also a politically tricky business. From overly cautious risk managers who patrol our words and publications for signs linking HIV, sexuality and pleasure to advocates who fear (justifiably in some cases) that the paltry amount of funding dribbling to HIV services will dry up completely if we let slip for a second the contention that the new treatments have made life worse for us all, suggestions that living with HIV can be pleasurable and anything but a litany of suffering and fears can be met with fierce opposition, and accusations of recklessness, inhumanity, or, worse yet, membership of the middle classes. Many of these attacks are mounted from within the HIV sector, where there sometimes appears to be a sort of consensus that it is the hardest hit, the most affected, who need to be represented as typical of the contemporary experience of living with HIV . . . The contrast with the rhetoric of the PLWHA movement in the early and mid 90s with that of today is so stark that you have to wonder why we were ever so misguided as to

vigorously oppose use of terms such as "victim" and "sufferer," and why we collectively invested so much in producing positive representations of people with HIV—in writing, art, photography, and other forms of communication.[30]

Brotherton provides a succinct analysis of a political climate in which "it is more and more necessary to make a case for excessive disadvantage in order to get even the most basic services." He explains how this makes it "harder and harder to speak of aspirations for the happiness of people with HIV, or to represent the possibility of pleasure in our lives." "But," he asks, "what does this do for people's sense of hope?"[31]

Brotherton frames the situation as a problem of articulating "everyday pleasures" in a context where almost half of the HIV-positive population lives in poverty and pleasure itself "is increasingly defined in terms of consumption."[32] His analysis shares themes with the columnist Brad Johnston's article, published in 1998 by the *Sydney Star Observer*, "Got the virus? Get the lifestyle."[33] Johnston recounts with a certain melancholy the styles of practice that developed "when the sense of crisis still necessitated action but humor was required to prevent exhaustion." He remembers a T-shirt "worn around town several years ago" that read "It's a virus, not a lifestyle." He goes on to ponder the new set of relations through which HIV identity was getting articulated in 1998—those of the pharmaceutical market. "Now that the sense of crisis has been reduced to a sense of responsibility, who needs it? The humor still exists, but only in its irony. After all, when even the most sophisticated tests can't detect the virus in your body, all you have left is a lifestyle."[34] Johnston's article is a wry comment on how marketing practices had begun to saturate the HIV imaginary. He even exploits the uneasy proximity of AIDS education and advertising genres, taunting "brand loyalty's a much more appealing concept than compliance, don't you think?" But his piece also reflects the real quandary and political despondency that the Protease Moment induced. How to conceive HIV politics, Johnston implies, when the fiction of a unitary biological essence at the basis of identity has apparently been erased, and when multinational corporations largely control the means of representation? How do we imagine collective futures when the practice of fighting AIDS has been reduced to a question of personal responsibility, consumer choice, and medical compliance and when people need to define their lives in terms other than disease? Appearing at a time when people were vacating the notion of HIV as central to their identity at a rate that was alarming for PLWHA organizations, many worried that the new forces mediating HIV were capable of rendering any viable mode of politics or social transformation undetectable.

Activating Sensibilities

It is possible to detect in Johnston's reference to being unable to detect the virus in the body a sense of disenchantment with notions of identity premised on the assumption of shared biology. Exhausted by the experience of the crisis and challenged by the many forms of experience that proved exception to its rule, the category of HIV identity no longer seemed sufficient for encompassing the modes of relation or identification that those whose lives had been affected by the epidemic saw themselves inhabiting or projecting into the future. The release of cumulative pressure from the crisis—precipitated, in part, by the arrival of new treatments—saw many wishing to define their lives in terms other than HIV. Nor should the effect on gay cultural formations generally be underestimated: in the introduction I described the waning interest in "community" structures that had previously and ecstatically proliferated in the otherwise bleak 1990s. As medical regimes rendered HIV experience private in new and constrictive ways, and as gay and HIV identity rebounded from the significant changes in orientation, intensity, and cohesion conferred by the Protease Moment, a need arose to find new ways of conceptualizing social agency and viability that looked not to what we *were*, but to how we live. This is why Brotherton and Johnston express such an ambivalent relation to consumption: they want to conceive a shared ground of experience that holds more promise than the limited alternatives of pathologized identity and the market.[35]

Some encouragement on this count may be taken from that well-worn policy phrase, "communities affected by HIV/AIDS." The allusion here to structures of affect—so mundane it often escapes notice—may offer a better frame than that of identity based on sexuality or serostatus when it comes to comprehending the forms of sociability, relation, and identification that have grown out of practices of responding to AIDS. I take *affect* here to refer not just to the structures of feeling arising from participation in specific social and cultural practices or historical conditions, but to the accumulation and cultivation of specific capacities—powers to move and to be moved. It evokes a sense of the passionate preconditions of social movements. Nor do I think it necessary or even possible to hold that the structures of feeling produced within particular historical conditions are uniform or evenly experienced—as Rosalyn Diprose has argued, community *lives from* difference, and bodies get passionate and sensibilities take shape through exposure to other bodies.[36] How this takes place—and according to which social technologies—is a matter for specific inquiry. But by shifting our attention to questions of affect and the social cultivation of sensibilities—to how different groups have been and are affected by the social technologies of AIDS, and how these effects provide in turn *a basis* for the formation of different sociabilities—it may be possible to approach a better understanding of the distinctive parameters and capacities for response at a given moment *without* having to psychologize individuals and *with* reference to the broad social and cultural structures within which subjects conduct their lives and experience them as meaningful.[37] This sort of inquiry becomes possible by looking at the cultural objects such groups consume, produce, and invest with particular meaning, and the description and analysis of significant examples and processes. Rather than depicting a trajectory of inevitable complacency and withdrawal (from HIV awareness), this approach asks about the conditions within which specific affects arise—their qualities and potential.

It is interesting in this regard that, just as Johnston expresses dismay at the prospect of imagining social continuity and political affectivity in the aftermath of the Vancouver conference, he reaches almost instinctively for a cultural style or structure of affect that is distinctive to homosexual communities. He mentions it explicitly—it is lodged right there between compliance and consumption—but in fact his whole article is a performance of it, and this works to bring a certain sort of public into being. Irony has a bad name these days—it is liable to be associated with exclusivity, faddishness, or elitism. But this perspective dismisses too quickly the relations that specific forms of irony—in this case, camp—enable. As a way of consuming cultural texts and performing them, camp has a long and expansive social history associated especially with gay experience but gaining a broader significance and utility in the context of popular or mass consumer culture. I want to approach it both as an embodied sensibility that (in this capacity) gestures toward more viable ways of conceptualizing social agency than notions of inner essence or identity *and* as a cultural repertoire that has had *specific* efficacy for negotiating the promises and indignities of antiviral medical regimes. I say "more viable," because these conceptualizations can be used to evoke a sense of identity based not on inner sameness or absolute continuity but on learned practices of performance, identification, recontextualization, interaction, differentiation, and response—in other words, living histories of cultural consumption and production. And efficacious, in that camp's historic proficiency at negotiating cultural authority has been put to new and unanticipated uses transforming the regimes of private consumption I have described under the Protease Moment.

In an earlier version of this analysis I noted the camp format of a treatment resource produced in 1997 by the AIDS Council of New South Wales. Released at the height of antiviral enthusiasm, the booklet adopts a "laundry detergent" aesthetic, employing garish colors and "bursts" (textual graphics to emphasize a product's bargain features) to declare "NOW more choices than ever before!"[38] I found this textual style intriguing, but left the question of what it might be doing unexplored. It seemed more a cultural quirk—a detail adding aesthetic appeal— than a choice bearing any particular health effects. Michael Hurley has also observed the existence of a "particular kind of campy humor" in community-based HIV treatment media, which cater to a PLWHA culture "that is simultaneously irreverent, and takes treatment knowledge seriously."[39] He makes a more considered case for the significance of this style, arguing that it sets up a productive tension with much of the written content, without which "the readability of [*Positive Living*] would change significantly."[40] Hurley's notion of HIV treatments media as "one of the primary ways a public, quasi-clinical space, largely controlled by the affected communities, is kept open" provides a useful lead into the operations of camp and their effectiveness in this context.[41] Specifically, camp negotiates reading positions for readers that allow them to bring their less-than-ideal experiences of treatment into articulation with the idealized narratives of capitalized medicine.[42]

Why should this matter? Partly as a point of contrast to the rational individualism that dominates professional discourses in the field. As a cultural style, camp relies on accumulated histories of practice and usage that are not predictable or universally shared, but specifically practiced and deployed. By contrast, health specialists tend to view education in terms of the straightforward delivery of fixed information or messages. As Hurley says of this discourse: "It is the content of the campaign advertisement that is seen as the primary determinant of meaning (a message is transmitted) rather than either the medium itself or a combination of both being involved interactively in the creation of public discourses between already linked networks. The reader is conceived as an individualized, passive recipient of a message and the media are transmitters rather than key players in the cultural narration of treatments and living with HIV."[43] Missing from this picture, as Hurley argues, is any sense of the social life of cultural forms. Textual style is treated as a colorful method of program delivery, rather than a specific exercise in engagement. Style matters only to the extent that it enhances the appeal of a static entity (the message) and facilitates its smooth transmission to the greatest number of people in the target group. Questions of cultural appropriateness, when they feature at all, treat the culture as a market rather than a scene of collective elaboration. They pertain to the "saleability" of the message in terms of its graphic or linguistic appeal. In some public health regimes, the individual's social and cultural attributes are as likely to be treated as a factor that must be controlled for the purposes of rigorous evaluation. The result, not surprisingly, is the production of interventions that work at the level of the rational unitary subject—though frequently in the most bland or instrumental of terms.[44] The message, in effect, becomes a drug.

One of the main points here is that even the agency of drugs is not limited to the terms suggested by controlled evaluation.[45] Drugs interact with particular assemblages and practices to produce their effects (which in the case of antiretroviral drugs may include longer life spans, changed apprehensions of AIDS, new modes of subjectification, and even the proliferation of new organisms: drug-resistant virus). Here, meaning and effect are understood, not as transmitted, but as produced through the interaction of various phenomena—specific interventions, figurations of media, practices, and bodies of memory. It is quite impossible to contain "effect" to the bounds of the individual body or a set time frame. In HIV education, too, meaning and effect entail these interdependencies. As Cindy Patton has argued with respect to safe sex, learning is not a simple matter of reading texts. Texts are taken up within particular matrixes of sexual participation and cultures of consumption that affect meaning, response, and responsiveness. Countering the educational assumption that language transparently communicates, Patton introduces the notion of *sexual vernacular* which she identifies as a matter of context, participation, observation, and modes of reading: "Understanding how a vernacular works requires identifying how values and concepts about sexuality and sexual practice have been effected within a community or micronetwork. The mediated and situated aspects of these symbolic processes—whether they are rap songs, dirty jokes, girl talk, how-to books—are the material templates for extending sex that saves our lives."[46] As Patton suggests, there is a necessary interactivity between texts and embodied styles of consumption, suggesting that health promotion could be understood as an exercise in cultivating specific sociabilities and embodied capacities by finding pertinent modes of address and intervention. Such a framework would seek to recognize how styles of address are interactively consequential, activating cultural memory and practice as resources in projects of self- and other-transformation.

The cultural resource I am interested in here is camp, which should be understood not only as a feature of certain texts and cultural objects, but also as a way of consuming texts and objects, which in turn has fashioned modes of producing cultural texts and objects. It has long been associated with homosexual subcultural tastes and styles, where the adulation of certain Hollywood film stars, texts, and other cultural objects resonated with the everyday experience of gender, sexual, and embodied incongruity and oppression, to produce a variety of nonliteral and parodic modes of reading, performance, humor, and sentiment.[47] In the context of twentieth-century consumer culture, camp gained a wider cultural resonance, where the pleasure taken in theatricality, the incongruous, and self-parody provided a popular way of negotiating the rapid turnover of cultural styles and a certain maneuverability with regard to regimes of taste.[48] Apart from its obvious place in a highly visible urban gay culture, camp has enjoyed a particular significance in Australian culture in terms of mediating relationships between the suburban and the metropolitan, as well as between the local and a British "parent" culture, where its revalorization of "bad taste" has prompted a range of popular cultural and iconic artifacts and personalities—from Dame Edna Everage and *Kath & Kim* (TV series) to *Muriel's Wedding* (P. J. Hogan, dir., 1994) and the films of Baz Luhrmann. It has also been used in critical parodies of the racism of white Australian ideology.[49] I am promoting camp here not (only) as a style that is "culturally appropriate" for this particular target audience, but as a specific affect, with specific histories, specific attributes, and specific potential. Clearly camp is going to jar or clash with some audients (proponents of an American-style, gay identity-politics spring first to mind.)[50] But the alternative to the specific proposal of affects in cultural pedagogy is to revert to a generic and affectless notion of transparent communication. Nor am I suggesting that camp is suitable for all HIV interventions.[51] The point is that it triggers a particular range of reader responses that might be considered when devising pedagogies. Like other embodied capacities, camp is learned and cultivated—not simply the natural *property* of bodies. Andrew Ross provides a useful handle on this in his essay title "Uses of Camp."[52] The challenge, as Sasha Torres has argued, is to appreciate how different bodies are transformed by these uses—to figure the difference that particular uses make for each other.[53]

In her analysis of camp and death, Caryl Flinn cites David Roman's contention that "the only way contemporary camp can exist is nostalgically, as a fleeting retreat into what he calls a 'pre-AIDS moment.' "[54] Given the use of camp in the tactics of ACT UP and queer theory, I don't find this claim entirely convincing. But it does raise the question of camp's relationship with the past. Camp might be thought to bear a reinvigorating relationship with the past. Andrew Ross, for his part, depicts camp as a scrounger through history's detritus and waste, creating a sort of "surplus value" out of outmoded and degraded cultural forms—where the only prerequisite for camp recuperation seems to be that the cultural form in question is a form "in decline."[55] In this regard, camp might be thought to rest on a certain degree of nostalgia. But while camp bears a fond relationship with the past, it does not retreat into the past entirely or brandish it as a law. As Flinn writes, "Camp might be said to function as a kind of *ironic* nostalgia, unlike more conventional forms of nostalgia, which mandate a much more earnest consumption of texts."[56] This does not preclude the existence of strong affect in camp's disposition toward the past. Susan Sontag calls camp a "tender feeling," and this sentiment might also be thought to frame camp's orientation to the future.[57] Arguing against the construction of camp as mere cynicism, for example, Eve Sedgwick finds in camp "a gayer and more spacious angle of view," which she explains by comparing it to "kitsch"— understood as cynical laughter at someone else's bad taste:

> Unlike kitsch-attribution, then, camp-recognition doesn't ask, "What kind of debased creature could possibly be the right audience for this spectacle?" Instead, it says *what if*: What if the right audience for this were exactly me? What if, for instance, the resistant, oblique, tangential investments of attention and attraction that I am able to bring to this spectacle are actually uncannily responsive to the resistant, oblique, tangential investments of the person, or of some of the people, who created it? And what if, furthermore, others whom I don't know or recognize can see it from the same "perverse" angle? Unlike kitsch-attribution, the sensibility of camp-recognition always sees that it is dealing in reader relations and projective fantasy (projective though not infrequently true) about the spaces and practices of cultural production.[58]

So while both kitsch and camp trade on a gap, a lag, a distance between subject and object, production and consumption, camp treats this as a relation—and more, as a hopeful relation. It projects, not a future self— but future relations. And this projection invests the unavoidable difference between subject and object, consumption and production, with generosity and open possibility. This is the sociability of camp. "Generous because it acknowledges (unlike kitsch) that its perceptions are also creations."[59]

Given its early detection in urban gay communities, camp was unavoidably implicated in the practices of responding to the AIDS epidemic. This happened less by design than because it was one of the cultural resources distinctive of, and existent within, gay culture. Writing on the workings of early Australian AIDS education initiatives, Gary Dowsett describes how "a safe sex culture creates an overarching discursive 'hum' that attracts gay men by situating safe sex within collectively defined and recognised activities and meanings. Keeping the momentum of that 'hum' going; renewing and re-presenting its message; amplifying its inclusivity; this has become the ongoing work of gay and community-based prevention interventions."[60] He is referring to the work that took place around politico-cultural events like the Sydney Gay and Lesbian Mardi Gras, which included not only safe sex poster campaigns but also activities such as mass condom distribution, musical performances, floats in the parade, and educators donning drag to act as "Safe Sex Sluts," and incorporated the work of community leaders, entertainers, gay media, and their publics. In terms of safe sex, these activities were associated with an unprecedented level of behavior change. But a decade later the salience of such events is in question, and the inability of poster campaigns to change individuals' behavior in direct and linear ways is sometimes cited as evidence of the failure of the entire community-based response. In such circumstances it seems particularly important to appreciate the intercorporeal dimensions of this "hum." In particular, rather than thinking of the HIV response as a question of bringing the body, understood as the site of a "reactive, undisciplined sensuality," under the control of a rational, informed mind, we might consider it as participant in processes of "experimentally *cultivated* responsiveness"—cultivated in interaction with other bodies.[61] This is to frame HIV responsiveness as something that requires apparatuses of public exchange. Such a perspective envisages interventions that seek to activate "collectively defined and recognised activities and meanings."[62] And it calls for active and participative practices of evaluation, where the question becomes, not just whether the intervention has produced the intended outcome—but the more open and responsible question of what embodied capacities, attributes, responses is it producing?

It's just such a "hum" that events like the *Wheel of Misfortune* aim to recreate when they opt for a format that is "part educative intervention, part peer support, and part good night out."[63] But rather than suggesting that this "hum" is just the generic "hum" of building social capital, I want to be more specific about it and examine how it works and what it might be doing.

The Wheel of Misfortune

The *Wheel of Misfortune* was set up in response to a reported desire for clear and accessible information around treatment side effects.[64] But while it and similar community treatment forums purport to cater to a simple deficit in information, their *style* of response also produces new contexts and capacities for engaging with medical knowledge and challenging its exclusions. This is particularly important when you consider that normative conventions of medical propriety are actually productive of some of the difficulties at hand. Many topics pertinent to HIV care—such as the experience of side effects, recreational drug use, or sex—become a matter of illegitimacy, difficult to articulate in the private space of the clinic. In these instances, medicine's appearance as a measure of social morality compromises its work as a practice of care. This can be the case despite (perhaps sometimes because of) the usual depiction of HIV patients as informed and sophisticated consumers.

The first thing to note about these treatment forums is their live-ness. Where most health-related frames catering to the epidemic at this time (such as mental health, substance abuse, self-esteem, and compliance) referred their solutions back onto the individual—rendering the problem a matter of individual dysfunction rather than collective concern—the *Wheel of Misfortune* works against this privatization of experience by bringing people together. This may sound trite, but its significance in relation to the isolation that can characterize HIV-positive experience is considerable. Second, the way it brings people together is fun and sociable. It's a night out. Before the start of the forums, Nurse Nancy and Vanessa mix with audience members to produce an atmosphere that is friendly, impudent, and funny. The way they do so remodels familiar arrangements of professional authority (see figure 5). Nurse Nancy, who wears a crisp white nurse's uniform (rather buxomly), entices individuals and groups of audience members to participate in her "community survey." Since the early 1990s, the practice of HIV surveying has been a perennial feature of gay events in Australia, where the prospect of being invited to fill in a lengthy survey about the most intimate details of one's sexual activities is sometimes a more likely prospect than participating in any such activities. Nurse Nancy was created in response to this feature of gay social life, first seen administering mock questionnaires at dance parties in 1996 to send up "scientific/educational pomposity."[65] The ingenuity of her character is how she stages scientific authority as performance. Pleasure and titillation are shown as suffusing familiar knowledge practices, rather than being extraneous to the knowledge relation. At the forum I attended, Nurse Nancy canvassed participants

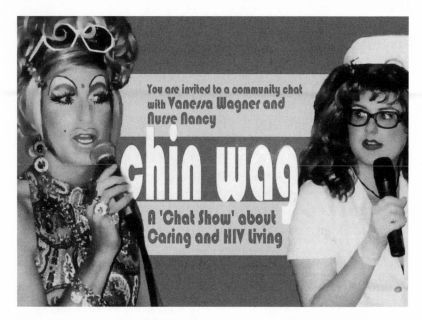

Fig. 5. Vanessa Wagner and Nurse Nancy from the *Wheel of Misfortune.*
Courtesy of the National Association of People with AIDS, Australia.

with questions like: "What are you on tonight?" "What's your favorite side effect?" "How are you being 'serviced' locally?" As well as muddling moral distinctions between the licit and the illicit, pleasure and discomfort, this encourages a level of humorous discussion around topics not generally the subject of polite social or easy clinical discourse. From the recreational use of drugs, to tensions in local service provision, it creates a zone of permission and encourages a level of impudence among participants that is entirely necessary for contending with the debilitating conditions of privacy produced around HIV-positive experience.

Two devices used during the show are specifically employed to contend these vectors of privatization. The selling point of Nurse Nancy's style of research is that she delivers her findings on the night. This raises issues that might otherwise remain covered, comically and seriously, without attributing them to individual authors. Also, an obscenely decorated "box" is passed around to deliver anonymous questions from the floor to the expert panel. Both these devices are attuned to the individual risks and collective promises of disclosure—the transformation of "dirty" private secrets into matters of public exchange. They operate in the knowledge that producing viability for HIV bodies requires challenges, however local, to the terms of public discourse. But they also operate in an awareness that such disclosure can put individuals at the risk of public censure. If contemporary modes of power work by making specifically embodied concerns exemplary of personal moral failure, then these devices go some way in working against this dynamic, raising such experiences as a matter of public elaboration, not immediately referable to a particular personality. So when Nurse Nancy lists "the drugs people are on tonight" (a list that will include alcohol, marijuana, antiretrovirals, party drugs, and so on), she is not simply relaying facts or creating a stir. She is acting on the terms of public exchange. She is producing, however provisionally, a different climate for public discourse and disclosure.[66]

Since the introduction of HAART, people with HIV have had to find ways of resisting the value accorded medical knowledge at the scene of clinical practice, so that an evaluation of treatment can emerge in the patient's terms. In this time, "quality of life" has emerged as an abstract, usable concept by means of which PLWHA have forced some recognition of the practicalities of consuming medicine.[67] It has framed discussions of side effects, body shape, treatment fatigue, and broader concerns, serving to withstand the overbearing emphasis on compliance. "Quality of life" clears a space in which a critique of HAART (in terms of the broader circumstances of life) can be made and entertained, serving as a useful device for wedging the patient's world further into the exchange. While there have been attempts to objectively determine measures of quality of life, the usefulness of the term in this context resides in the impossibility of determining a life's quality without reference to the patient's subjective evaluation of his or her circumstances. It arises as a theme when the worth of a medical solution is in dispute, giving patients some leverage in the construction of problems and solutions.

Camp does similar work in these forums, though perhaps in a more entertaining and collaborative way. It places an entertainment value on the incongruity between subjective experience and medical ideality, encouraging the articulation of normally subjugated experiences and projecting a background of collective concern that emboldens shared capacities for disclosure. Vanessa herself embodies this incongruity, mixing the style of exaggerated 1960s suburban housewife with the demands of social activism and contemporary glamour. Vanessa adopts a "sensible shoes" approach to matters of social and political conscience, but the other voice operating in her performance is one that affirms the realities of pleasure and gratification. No stranger to getting "carried away" with things, she manages to come across in turn as prim, pragmatic, ethical, and hedonic—a spectacular embodiment of the awkward and always incomplete process of reconciling comfort, safety, concern, and glamour. In her questions and interactions with the expert panel, Vanessa stages the authority that her guests (and herself) represent as interjectable and incomplete. She frequently makes reference to her experience as an HIV-positive gay man, acting as a sort of "fall guy" (fall gal?) to confront medical seriousness with the day-to-day practicalities of life with the virus. Participants are not just being entertained here. They are witnessing the articulation of experiences of consumption back onto the spaces of medical production and knowledge.

Camp's ability to negotiate hierarchies of taste is useful here, where most of the experience in question involves the unruly, the protuberant, or the abject body. Camp's fascination with bodily excess—what Caryl Flinn describes as "the disunified body, the funny body that doesn't quite fit with itself"—helps to elicit a comic posture on attributes and experiences deemed to threaten bodily integrity and closure, rendering them a source (and potential target) of laughter.[68] In this respect, camp shares qualities with the body of grotesque realism—the material, defecating, abject body that momentarily disrupts conventional boundaries with its unwholesome and exuberant flesh.[69] The *Wheel of Misfortune* itself plays on this disruption: the experience of side effects puncturing the narrative of fame, fortune, and commercial self-realization implicit in the format. The invocation of fortune and chance in the title of the format similarly casts the experience of side effects in terms of accident and the luck of the draw, which counters the sense in which such effects can materialize as a reflection of personal moral worth. When the wheel is spun, the question of which side effect will come up is the matter of suspense. Bitterly parodying the experience of "winning the game," this format replicates in miniature the intense structures of hope and disappointment that accompanied the introduction of HAART for many PLWHA. The parody provides a degree of ironic distance from such an experience, which also serves to acknowledge the complications of feeling that attended the introduction of these medical commodities.

The question "what's your favorite side effect?" deploys camp in a similar fashion. Initially confrontational for people who have lived through some of the indignities of HIV treatment, the question provides an affective handle with which to configure the experience for public elaboration. It enables the voicing of a consumer perspective on the experience of medicine. "Power-*mincing* to the toilet!" was the answer supplied by one participant the night I attended. I want to dwell on this image for a moment because it is not simply making fun of an awful situation. Nor is my claim that camp somehow magically transcends such bodies and experiences, but that it exposes them, and exposes them as problematic. If, in his analysis of camp, Andrew Ross frames camp as a sort of elitist solution to the assault on hierarchies of taste that occurred in the context of 1960s mass culture (he calls it "cultural slumming where others would feel less comfortable"), we can see that here this ability to maneuver between the "high" and "low" without relinquishing a claim on cultural dignity is quite important.[70] When it is the conventions of healthy decorum that are responsible for rendering one's experience negligible, the capacity to violate standards of good taste while preserving amicable relations is crucial. Here the low is recuperated as a source of public elaboration, without denying its social materiality as distasteful or unpleasant. "Power-mincing to the toilet" is such an evocative instance of camp because it references the conditions that compound the indignity of this situation—the glamour value of health regimes and their insinuation with gender. It forces attention onto the body, hoping to test and refigure the limits of shame, disgust, and empathy. Camp's ability (which Richard Dyer notes in his discussion of the gay fascination with Judy Garland) to "hold together qualities that are elsewhere felt as antithetical: theatricality and authenticity . . . intensity and irony, a fierce assertion of extreme feeling with a deprecating sense of its absurdity" is important here.[71] The experience is posed as absurd, and intense, but also as contingent—demanding better drugs, better strategies, and better conditions of materialization.

This raises the question of the sort of laughter that camp trades on and the promise of its sometimes ruthless debasement of the self (or other).

Let me give another example. In "Lipodysphoria: A Growing Concern," Brad Johnston takes the changes to HIV-positive political identity attending the introduction of HAART as his subject.[72] He refers to the "sense of outrage and scope for complaint" that characterized HIV speaking positions in the early 1990s, suggesting these have "succumbed to the relentless progress of medical treatment." For this reason, he jokes, "lipodystrophy is a godsend." He refers here to the unusual condition of fat redistribution associated with the use of treatment: "Just when we'd resigned ourselves to the fact that our dramatic exit was on indefinite hold . . . we're presented with something that strikes at the very heart of contemporary Western insecurity—body image. It does sound monumentally trivial doesn't it? Your typical queen's shallow hysteria. Think about the countless PLWHA in developing nations who don't even have access to treatment! Well, I might have some time to do that if I weren't so preoccupied with the small, indecisive mound which has appeared above my waistband." Johnston draws out the striking ambiguities of medical security. The population of PLWHA have had to "resign themselves" to the uncertainty of life, while "lipo doesn't have the reassuring finality of death." It's not death, meanwhile, but *appearance* that "strikes at the very heart of contemporary Western insecurity." Johnston's response is to propose an erotic revaluation of pathology. Reminding his audience that "one man's fear is another man's fetish," he plays on the condition's nickname "buffalo hump" to propose, "It's a simple matter of embracing your inner aesthete": "With enough media coverage and community support we can really put the ox back into Oxford Street—the annual Dance With Wolves, Stampede every Sunday night at the Barracks, perhaps a monthly affair at the Den simply called Hump."

Johnston isn't just being camp here. He seems to be parodying the camp position that would have everything available to recontextualization at the whim of postmodern aesthetes. There's almost a sense that camp has been pushed to its limits, that its tactics have been exhausted in a way that appears to confirm David Roman's contention that "the only way contemporary camp can exist is nostalgically, as a fleeting retreat into a 'pre-AIDS' moment."[73] It's as though camp sensibilities can't quite address the gravity of the situation. This sense is compounded in an uncharacteristic moment of moral seriousness from Johnston in the final paragraph: "Okay, I know, I'm pushing it. Lipo doesn't have the reassuring finality of death, nor does it elicit the sympathy of debilitation. It just gnaws away at the rawest of nerves and shakes the foundations of our newly built confidence. Then again, there's nothing like a little cosmetic adversity to rally the troops. Complacency might very well be endangered. Could this be the call to re-gay the epidemic?" In this hilarious about-turn, Johnston configures for public elaboration a condition whose shame is otherwise produced as mandatory. He approaches lipodystrophy as a question of *how problems come to matter for people*, using camp humor to dramatize and unsettle such practices of mattering. But part of the problem that is being confronted here is precisely the exhaustion of camp: the systematic erasure of queer energies and labor in medical accounts of responding to the epidemic. In the end, we are almost seduced into a posture of medical reality. To my knowledge, this is the only discussion of lipodystrophy to have appeared in the Sydney gay press. For the camp reader, then, the last paragraph's "what if?" is also deadly serious.

Conclusion

The analysis of camp that I have developed in this chapter is intended to illustrate how one embodied style (which exists as part of the embodied repertoire of a group that has been significantly impacted by the HIV epidemic) has come in useful for contesting some of the less endurable forms of privatization and individualization that inhere in the discourse of compliance. As a mode of consuming texts and artifacts, camp sensibility can be understood to have entered into an innovative articulation with competing bodily priorities. Where the discourse of compliance renders certain unexpected or unwanted effects of drugs as a matter of individual responsibility and private shame, this embodied style has been actively and usefully deployed to throw these matters up for public consideration, elaboration, and concern. This in turn has provided more inhabitable contexts within which decisions about well-being and bodily experience might be made, and in which different priorities around the body are more openly aired and contested. The effect, I would argue, is to enable more responsive forms of care.

A focus on embodied sensibilities may provide a more promising and user-friendly frame for understanding the possibilities of connection and responsiveness around health problems than that which is constrained by the demands of selfsame identity. In the context of antiretroviral politics, for example, there is something crucial to recognize in the emergence of forms of global political conscience that, in Gregory Palast's words, marred Al Gore's presidential campaign trail by "attracting packs of enraged homosexuals who hollered about his killing more Africans than Michael Caine in *Zulu*."[74] Such (otherwise) unlikely political connections and points of contact disrupt the logic that would have one set of political and cultural subjectifications occurring "at the expense of" another. By conceiving how one embodied sensibility provides connective interfaces with, and thus enlivens, differently situated problems, we can develop a more dynamic approach to public health that is nonetheless attentive to embodied specificity. Camp is obviously not the only form of active consumption that recontextualizes the meanings and effects of medical discourse. The connective possibilities of active consumption are grounded in the cultural specificities of embodiment in any given situation.[75] Thus while camp could be considered specifically sensitized to the regulatory categories of sexuality—the public and private, shame and disgust—it is merely one example of how medical categories and imperatives have been productively reworked through irreverent pleasure and a distinct style of cultural consumption. The challenge for HIV and health activists is to work with the distinctive sensibilities and modes of embodiment of affective (and not just affected) communities.

6

EMBODIMENTS OF SAFETY

...

Eve Sedgwick says of Oscar Wilde's *The Picture of Dorian Gray* (1891) and Robert Louis Stevenson's *The Strange Case of Dr. Jekyll and Mr. Hyde* (1886) that "both books begin by looking like stories of erotic tensions between men, and end up as cautionary tales of solitary substance abusers."[1] Gay responses to AIDS have been forced to endure the same cultural narrative. Some years after the medical establishment declared HIV a chronic manageable illness, Melbourne's respectable daily treated its readers to the cartoon image of a decrepit skeleton, complete with fairy wings, guzzling pills as he staggers to the ground. The caption read "Party Animal" (see figure 6). The illustration accompanied an article, "Dancing with Death," that accounted for what was in fact a small rise in HIV infections as follows:

> Many will not be surprised. Recent surveys in Sydney and Melbourne have shown a greater incidence of sex without condoms. Health professionals believe it is not just casual unsafe sex, but problems with people getting into relationships and having unsafe sex before both partners are tested.
>
> More to the point, however, a nexus has been found between drug use—ecstasy and speed, inextricably linked to the dance-party circuit—and unsafe sex. Young gay men are taking risks because—like other young men—they believe they are indestructible. In this case, however, gay men have had their minds altered by illicit drugs, and they assume the new protease inhibitor drug combinations will save them.
>
> Young gay men looking for a way to belong join the dance-party circuit and feel the peer pressure to over-indulge in drugs, which in turn impair their judgment over risk-taking behaviour.[2]

Steve Dow treads a well-worn narrative path here. His depiction of gay men "partying on as though illicit drugs will make them forget the world outside, while prescription drugs will save them from the threat of the virus" is the very image of technological and consumptive excess. Linked to the Internet, to drugs, and to a commercial scene, gay men are typified as self-destructive narcissists, technologically fixated, partying themselves to death.[3] Dow even prefaces his account by alluding to its cultural availability: "Many will not be surprised." Surprise is indeed misplaced, but not for the reasons the author would have us confirm. The extraordinary levels of behavior change sustained in the first decades of the epidemic were adopted in response to a far more threatening prognosis. Gay men are no longer quite "dancing with death," but "with chronic manageable illness" (an epigraph that admittedly lacks punch). I don't mean here to recommend the acquisition of chronic illness, simply to observe that, given these changed conditions, some revaluation of risk is comprehensible—to be expected, even. But rather than give this point any serious consideration, commentators around the world preferred to depict gay men as self-consumed hedonists who had forgotten the moral lessons of AIDS. Drugs featured heavily in this alchemy of moral instruction. The sense of security inspired by the new therapies was said to be unwarranted and false—at least when it came to sex. Gay men were using recreational drugs said to cause risk by reducing sexual inhibitions and enhancing the libido. U.S. pharmaceutical companies were accused of encouraging risk in glitzy drug advertisements that glamorized the lives of people with HIV. And prevention specialists focused their attention on whether fear was an effective motivator. By all accounts, gay men were now to be treated as the ultimate "cultural dopes."

Perhaps a more edifying story is the remarkable modification of sexual and drug practices sustained by those at risk, which has taken place *with* reference to a culture of pleasure, and largely withstanding conservative structures of authority and practice. "At the very moment when freedom from risk was becoming a dominant social promise, AIDS education had the task of pioneering entirely new protocols of safety," as Andrew Ross puts it.[4] But this is not a story that we are likely to hear in contemporary publics, precisely because it would involve an account of pleasures that exceed normative forms. It is virtually impossible to speak of the

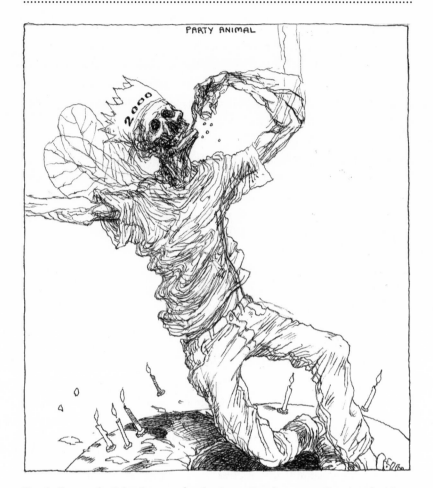

Fig. 6. Cartoon by John Spooner for the *Age*, 4 October 2000. Reprinted with the permission of John Spooner and the *Age*.

pleasure of illicit drugs, for instance, in any forum that considers itself public or healthy. In some of the early work on moral panic, Jock Young argued that this is because of the media's assumption of a consensual ideology at the base of its address (and not just the random ignorance of journalists).[5] Young describes the drug taker as the "deviant *par excellence*" because the behavior appears to dodge the norms of hard work, family life, and industrious consumption that maintain the moral citizen. Pleasures are the just reward for hard work, in this imaginary, and those that are taken outside this moral structure must appear as a scandal or else not real pleasure at all. The excitement that surrounds these undeserved pleasures (and contributes to the sale of a great number of newspapers) must therefore be tempered with just the right amount of moral indignation to confirm people's adherence to "culturally approved goals" and "normatively sanctioned means," according to Young.[6] The drug user is never happy in the end.

Young's account sheds light on the depiction of the Party Animal—though here it is as much homosexuality as drug use that bears the brunt of public indignation. As HIV enters a new, more manageable phase, illicit drugs appear to have taken up the slack in the public narrative of just desserts that has come to haunt gay life. Here, AIDS is cast as an opportunity for growing up—the crisis gay men had to have. The targets of concern are always young (though in Australia most new infections take place among men aged thirty and over) such that we can't be sure whether the cautionary tale is about HIV transmission or the perils of failing to settle down to normal (heterosexual) responsibilities. Hence the infantilizing of the party animal (the fairy wings, candles, and party hat). What's more, the moral occasion tends to take precedence over effective communication of the realities of HIV risk. Thus while Dow makes reference to the fact that many (in Australia, almost half of) new infections occur as an effect of placing too much faith in the ostensible security of conjugal intimacy, note how quickly this fact is subordinated to the thrust of the primary narrative. ("More to the point . . . a nexus has been found between drug use . . . and unsafe sex." What "point" makes this nexus more significant exactly?) In the end, it doesn't actually matter whether the pills in the picture are viewed as therapeutic or recreational (and the shape of the bottle suggests they could be either): life or death, enjoyment or despair, it's all the same, a technological fix, for this doomed form of life. The Party Animal has failed to convert his consuming pleasure into normative currency. With their proximity to "other [normal] young men" noted, gay men are made to embody a cultural tendency viewed as latent and ubiquitous, but repudiated as other. Collapsing into (and as) the party boy, the Party Animal secures a more wholesome zone for those who aren't, in a horrible projection of *fin de millennium* decadence.

Illicit drugs have in fact always been part of the environment in which both risk and safety (with respect to HIV transmission) have been practiced.[7] Since the introduction of HAART, however, they have increasingly been cast in this more determinative role. This delivers both HIV *and* drug education to the custodians of public morality—in either the mode of moral condemnation (declaiming "abuse") or else corrective intervention (treating "addiction"). By positioning drugs as causative of HIV risk, these accounts present HIV as an outcome of personal acts of moral transgression. But HIV transmission has very little to do with the state of personalities and a lot to do with particular activities and relations between bodies. In this chapter I will offer an alternative account of what has worked in HIV prevention and drug education. My argument is that the achievements of these fields suggest the utility of a distinction between embodied ethics and normative morality—a distinction that has allowed health workers to articulate and engage the embodied pleasures of endangered groups, rather than deny them. Of course it makes a certain amount of intuitive sense that health interventions are most effective when phrased in terms of the values, media, and sources of authority that are respected by those they seek to address. But what complicates this task when the risk involves "illicit" activities (such as homosexuality or drug use) is that it is precisely the provision of this sort of material that is precluded by public morality.

Ethics and Technique

Though they have developed into distinct fields of practice and policy, both gay men's HIV education and harm reduction had as their initial conditions of possibility the highly moralized climate of the AIDS crisis. In these circumstances, these fields strategically adopted a "value-neutral" stance in the field of public policy. This involved a rhetorical distinction between *scientific facts* and *moral values*. When moral reactionaries condemned homosexuality, activists could appeal to the scientific fact that HIV could be prevented by the use of condoms. When conservatives objected to the institution of needle exchanges, practitioners could appeal to the public health objective of HIV prevention. Of course, these "rational" responses were also "moral" responses in fact. They claimed a moral entitlement to health for homosexuals, sex workers, drug users, and other marginalized subjects. Moreover, as Helen Keane argues with respect to the highly moralized arena of drug debate, "a view that drug use is neither right nor wrong is *not* neutral, but is itself a committed and critical standpoint."[8] Nevertheless, it remains the case that harm reduction and HIV prevention have made substantial gains by framing themselves in the rational and technical discourse of public health (as Keane argues).

At the same time, there is a sense that the failure to articulate a more open stance on pleasure leads to shortcomings in the position of harm reduction. For example, Stephen Mugford has argued that without any acknowledgement of the perceived benefits of pleasure, even the most hard-line antidrug campaigners are able to identify themselves as harm reductionists, on the basis of a supposedly neutral calculation of costs and benefits.[9] Within HIV prevention, John Ballard argues that one of the strengths of safe sex as an educational concept was that it was "sex-positive at a time of maximum stigmatisation of gay men."[10] And Pat O'Malley and Mariana Valverde point to the absence of pleasure as an explanation for drug use in harm-reduction education materials to argue that the "more or less explicit model of the subject deployed in harm minimization is that of the rational choice actor who will perform the felicity calculus."[11] Harm reduction is situated within a highly technical and rationalist framework that proposes the objective calculation of risks and harms, producing, for example, an "enormous amount of attention [to] the mechanics of drug administration."[12] However, I suggest that the technical aspects of safe practice are important precisely because they engage the bodily *hexis* of those at risk. In this sense, they are not neutral or divorced from the field of value, but culturally embodied and experimentally cultivated. Here is Marcel Mauss on techniques of the body: "The body is man's first and most natural instrument. Or more accurately, not to speak of instruments, man's first and most natural technical object, and at the same time technical means, is his body. . . . Before instrumental techniques there is the ensemble of techniques of the body. . . . The constant adaption to a physical, mechanical or chemical aim (e.g., when we drink) is pursued in a series of assembled actions, and assembled for the individual not by himself alone but by all his education, by the whole society to which he belongs, in the place he occupies in it."[13] Mauss notes cultural and historical as well as individual differences in styles of swimming, walking, giving birth (despite his masculinist language), eating, jumping, and having sex. It's in this sense that I claim that techniques and technologies are culturally embodied. They are not only (or not just) instrumental or mechanical means, but acquired, used, and cultivated within specific cultural fields and situations.

Now, one of the crucial innovations of both HIV education and harm reduction alike has been that, rather than holding out for disembodied ideas of the good, they have met people at the level of concrete embodied practice. This can be as simple as distributing technical devices such as condoms or clean syringes at critical moments so that people can do more safely what they were going to do anyway. Or it can take the form of a reflexive discussion of bodily situation and technique. The crucial thing at any rate is not the blanket reinforcement of abstract norms, but how certain techniques have been incorporated into bodily practices, situations, and styles. In the second and third volumes of *The History of Sexuality*, Michel Foucault seeks to open ethics up to a consideration of different modes of being. He makes a distinction between morality (which he understands as a system of universal rules and regulations) and ethics (which he frames as the practical techniques through which individuals and groups make themselves the subject of certain moral codes). Writing at the onset of the AIDS crisis, one of Foucault's concerns in this work is "how to adapt and direct the power exercised by medical, quasi-medical and moral experts in the time of the AIDS epidemic."[14] He is less concerned with the enforcement of any particular moral code therefore than the techniques and relations through which certain moral principles come to be enacted.

Foucault conceives the possibility in this work of what Jane Bennett calls an "experimentally *cultivated* responsiveness."[15] If his earlier work demonstrates the pervasiveness of socially imposed discipline, this later work suggests a slim margin of possibility between discipline imposed and practices of self-elaboration, yielding what Foucault calls "technologies of the self."[16] While for some this conjures individualistic images of mind over matter, it need not. Foucault merely casts the self as a "object of knowledge and field of action" to which one may bring a certain degree of care and attention.[17] He does not imagine that ethics lie entirely outside disciplinary structures, but rather that power is never entirely effective—that it is incomplete, and that by making this margin of error an object of conscious care and elaboration, it might be possible to devise new forms of subjectivity that contend the normative operations of power.[18] Foucault's ethics turn to pleasure to devise new modes of subjectivity that are less available to prevailing patterns of domination. In his subsequent work on "care of the self," he wants to conceive forms of care and self-relation that could pry themselves away from normative determinations where necessary, but retain some form of ethical stylization.[19]

There are echoes of this later work in Douglas Crimp's argument, made in the early days of the AIDS epidemic: "We were able to invent safe sex because we have always known that sex is not, in an epidemic or not, limited to penetrative sex. Our promiscuity taught us many things, not only about the pleasures of sex, but about the great multiplicity of those pleasures. It is that psychic preparation, that experimentation, that conscious work on our own sexualities that has allowed many of us to change our sexual behaviours—something that brutal 'behavioural therapies' tried unsuccessfully for over a century to force us to do—very quickly and very dramatically."[20] For Crimp, safe sex is an outgrowth of embodied improvisation.[21] The initial appearance of AIDS among gay men and drug users in the West gave rise to dogmatic calls for abstinence, monogamy, and quarantining.[22] These calls did not just come from moral reactionaries; they were the logical extension of prevailing mechanisms of public health and medical science.[23] They were premised, that is, on rationalities that positioned those at risk as objects of government, rather than subjects of their own care. Not only did endangered groups withstand these calls, but they also devised strategies that successfully prevented transmission without demanding a "return" to normative forms of sexual and corporeal life. Of course, these strategies did not develop in some political vacuum of "lived experience." They drew on existing techniques of comportment, and called on competing sources of moral and scientific authority to validate themselves as measures. But in an equally important sense, they installed a distinction between normative morality and embodied elaboration, and cast this distinction as a space of ethical possibility—upon which lives depended. In this respect, embodied practice is not simply something that prevention specialists have had to take into account when devising safe strategies. It has actively shaped the production and maintenance of such strategies.

The findings of social science certainly bear out a relation between embodied subjectivity and the strategies that have been successful with respect to HIV prevention. While gay men largely ignored the moral calls for abstinence and monogamy, between 1986 and 1996 there was an uptake of prevention strategies grounded in the embodied styles of those at risk, including the use of condoms for anal sex, an expansion of the sexual repertoire in terms of the adoption of relatively safe sexual practices, and, when HIV testing became common, negotiated safety (where regular partners of the same HIV status negotiate an agreement with respect to sex that happens inside and outside the relationship).[24] Not only did gay men and drug users choose some strategies and eschew others, but there is also evidence for the effectiveness of these strategies. As Susan Kippax and I have shown, the strategies that have been most successful have been those based on a mutually acceptable description of safety from the perspectives of official science and the embodied positions of those at risk. "Gay men, injecting drug users, and, to some degree, heterosexuals moved to make their practices safe—by modifying and building on them, not by abstaining from or eliminating them."[25] The picture of agency that emerges from these data is neither that of the self-knowing, decisional subject whose actions are the result of rational choice and disembodied control, nor the behavioral automaton that merely reproduces given norms, but rather something much more akin to embodied ethics. Safe practice is an outcome of embodied habits, cultural memory, and sedimented history; but it also depends, to some extent, on ethical improvisation and modification. In other words, the rhetorical distinction between *scientific facts* and *moral values* that framed early responses to the epidemic is only one part of the story. An active element in the midst of these categories is embodied culture.

Uses of Medicine

One of the advantages of recognizing embodied agency in the field of HIV has been how it elucidates the effect of medical technologies on prevention. When a decline in consistent condom use became apparent among gay men in the 1990s, many epidemiologists spoke of recidivism or noncompliance. Research that was more sensitive to the social contexts of gay sex was able to detect that gay men were using the medical technology of HIV testing to enable relatively safe, unprotected sex within regular relationships.[26] A number of gay men were discarding condoms for sex within seroconcordant regular relationships, but continued to use them within casual contexts. Australian educators responded to this finding by conducting specific education in order to make this strategy safer, termed "negotiated safety."[27] Since it is unreasonable to expect adult individuals not to inform and avail themselves of medical knowledge, the most feasible option open to educators seemed to be to make the existence of this practice known to affected individuals and enhance its safety. This involved conceding the relative efficacy of this strategy in terms of HIV prevention. While some decried this move as eroding the condom norm, negotiated safety can also be understood as an ethical response on the part of education agencies to the way this medical technology was being used within gay relations. What is important to recognize here is that this technology was being used in ways shaped by the cultural practices governing gay relations—and these are the practices with which gay education had to work. It was not simply a matter of providing scientific information on risk, but of attending to the concrete situation of gay relationships—their existence alongside and within a culture of casual sex. Educational campaigns addressed these circumstances by providing guidance on a number of strategies (HIV testing, open discussion, agreement on condom use outside the relationship) that would enhance the safety of these sexual and relational practices.

The introduction of HAART saw further changes to the sexual cultures of gay men—in particular rises in unprotected sex (though these rises were not necessarily accompanied immediately by increases in HIV infections).[28] Qualitative research conducted in 2000 identified the existence of a range of considered strategies other than condom use and negotiated safety in gay men's accounts of unprotected sex.[29] These included the use of viral load test results to estimate the risk of infection, withdrawal before ejaculation, disclosure of HIV status, and the adoption of an insertive or receptive position when engaging in unprotected anal intercourse, depending on HIV status. Subsequent quantitative analyses confirmed the use of these strategies to reduce risk among Sydney gay men.[30] When engaging in unprotected anal intercourse, HIV-negative men in casual encounters were more likely than not to adopt the insertive role, while HIV-positive men were more likely to be receptive. This finding was stronger in serodiscordant regular relationships in which sexual partners are more likely to share knowledge and understandings of viral load. When the behavior of the same men was examined when they used condoms, the pattern completely disappeared, and reciprocity returned. This suggests that sexual position was being selected strategically on the basis of HIV status and safety, and did not relate simply to personal preference for a particular sexual position.

Whatever the relative efficacy of these strategies, their existence contradicts the stereotype of the gay cultural dope that has haunted the Protease Moment. What seems to be the case is that the introduction of HAART provided the conditions of possibility for a limited process of revaluation of risk among gay men. It remains the case that a majority of gay men report using a condom in every instance of anal sex in a defined interval, but an expansion of relatively well-informed prevention ethics that do not equate with the condom ethic is also apparent.[31] This is not a picture of people throwing caution to the wind. It is a picture of gay men appropriating medical knowledge to craft a range of considered strategies that attempt to balance sex and the avoidance of risk. These strategies are not foolproof. But many of them are scientifically plausible on the basis of epidemiological evidence, indicating a relatively informed engagement with scientific and probabilistic reasoning in gay men's sexual accounts and practice. It is not at all clear that probabilistic reasoning is always appropriate for the purposes of HIV prevention (which always involves two or more people who may be bringing different assumptions to the encounter). But prevention specialists need to know what sexual subjects are doing in order to respond appropriately. These strategies adapt medicine to fit the cultural desires of subjects for pleasure and safety. What emerges is a field of complex evaluation that does not always rank long-term health over everyday desires for intimacy, sensuality, and pleasure.

The use of medicine within gay sexual repertoires raises a number of challenges for HIV educators, not least the challenge of enhancing the safety of these practices. This entails more than supplying people with scientific information about the risks of various practices and more than a celebration of agency. Upon the identification of the workings of medicine in gay sex, the field of HIV prevention in Australia became prolific with accounts of "sophisticated gay men making complex decisions to reduce risk." At times, these descriptions seemed to verge on a populist romanticism that celebrated every instance of gay men's appropriation of medicine as though it were inherently safe. We heard a lot about gay men's "cultures of care," for example, but comparatively little was offered in the way of empirical analysis of the shape of these cultures, or the practices of differentiation that went into ensuring care, or their concrete effects. Often one was left with the impression that all gay educators needed to do was provide a few scientific facts, trust gay men, and put all stock in lived cultures that were inherently resistant, subversive, communal, sophisticated, and safe. To some extent, these problems are inherent in the theories of everyday life upon which these analyses more or less explicitly draw.[32] The excess of process over structure is often regarded as cause for political celebration in itself, with little concern for how, concretely, such excess reworks the social field. But applied to the field of HIV prevention, these impressions become as good an argument as any for justifying the shortfalls that currently threaten to wind down education and research in the field of gay men's health promotion. After all, if gay culture is inherently well-informed and productive of non-problematic cultures of care, there is not much left for health educators to do. It seems to me that the reason for attending to embodied agency in the field of health promotion is not simply to celebrate the endlessly inventive practices of everyday life or sex (though well we might). It is to provide much-needed information about the cultural conditions in which particular dangers and possibilities—both social and physical— take shape. Some of these possibilities arise from the very practices of differentiation that are adopted to promote safety (such as those that discriminate between HIV-positive or HIV-negative sexual partners, or, as I will discuss later, between different forms of drug use). Health promoters need to monitor the cultural effects of these practices and discourses carefully and, when their effects become problematic, respond to them.

A Taste for Drugs

In an interview in 1984, Michel Foucault remarked on the cultural dimensions of drug use:

> M.F.   I think that drugs must become a part of our culture.
>
> Q.   As a pleasure?
>
> M.F.   As a pleasure. We have to study drugs. We have to experience drugs. We have to do *good* drugs that can produce very intense pleasure. I think this puritanism about drugs, which implies that you can either be for drugs or against drugs, is mistaken. Drugs have now become a part of our culture. Just as there is bad music and good music, there are bad drugs and good drugs. So we can't say we are "against" drugs any more than we can say we're "against" music.[33]

For some, these remarks will only serve as further evidence of the pathological personality behind this thinker's work. This is because drugs, no less than homosexuality or madness, are key operators in contemporary regimes of power and knowledge that confer upon everyone else except those linked to the practice "a power of irrefutable judgment" over them.[34] As Foucauldian scholars have shown so well, such regimes operate through strategic procedures of legitimation and delegitimation. In effect, the subjective account of the experience in question is denied any validity in the scheme of authorized knowledge that surrounds it, except insofar as it can be used to confirm the pathological status of the personality in question. Indeed, Foucault's remarks can be read as combating exactly this tendency in drug discourse. They amount to an argument for the cultivation of critical and subjective expertise in the field. Today Foucault would be accused of "condoning drug use," and the epistemological privilege of those who claim they know the truth about drugs (and those who use them) would be reiterated.

In fact, the charge of "condoning" a behavior always puts the authority in question in a juridical position with respect to the behavior. Apart from presuming the wrongness of the activity in the first place, this inevitably involves some suppression of the responsibility and freedom of those who would make themselves the subjects of such authority. As many have observed (usually with some frustration) it is precisely such a normative use of authority that Foucault sought, throughout his career, to refuse. But while Foucault generally resisted the pressure to use his position to tell people what they should do or how they should behave, this isn't exactly true of this passage, which makes a blatantly normative appeal. We have to experience drugs, he says. The advice is hardly equivocal. Should I take the author at his word here, and go out and take drugs indiscriminately? Or should I situate the authority of this text and make a decision for myself? Given the force of contemporary prohibitions around the positive articulation of drugs, it is almost impossible to occupy a docile relation to this text. In a sense, the passage performs the readerly relations it anticipates. These relations are continued in the remarks that follow. Thus, the advice to do drugs is quickly followed by a qualification in the realm of value. It's not just *any* drugs that are advised here, but "*good* drugs that can produce very intense pleasure." But beyond being pleasing, the criteria of value are not specified. Instead, an analogy with music is made: "Just as there is bad music and good music, there are bad drugs and good drugs." Foucault seems to be flagging the possibility of a politics of cultural value around drugs.

In his book on popular music, Simon Frith argues that aesthetic judgment is the very fabric of popular culture. The pleasure that one takes in music and other cultural forms is accumulated in the body as taste—through knowledge, experience, and training—such that it is experienced as deeply personal and innate. But it is also a means of distinction and social classification. Drawing on Pierre Bourdieu's argument that aesthetic discrimination is socially functional—that it displays social or class membership—Frith argues that "a similar use of accumulated knowledge and discriminatory skill is apparent in low cultural forms, and has the same hierarchical effect. Low culture, that is to say, generates its own capital—most obviously, perhaps, in those forms (such as dance club cultures) which are organised around exclusiveness, but equally significantly for the fans (precisely those people who have invested time and money in the accumulation of knowledge) of even the most inclusive forms."[35] Frith continues, "What I'm suggesting here is that people bring similar questions to high and low art, that their pleasures and satisfactions are rooted in similar analytic issues, similar ways of relating what they see or hear to how they think and feel. The differences between high and low emerge because these questions are embedded in different historical and material circumstances, and are therefore framed differently, and because the answers are related to different social situations, different patterns of sociability, different social needs."[36] This is not to say that power is absent from the terrain of cultural taste. On the contrary, every cultural field has its sources of authority and evaluative principles, and these exist in a relation of tension, struggle, and play. As Frith contends, "Part of the pleasure of popular culture is talking about it; part of its meaning is this talk, talk which is run through with value judgments. To be engaged with popular culture is to be discriminating, whether judging the merits of a football team's backs or an afternoon's soap plots."[37] In other words, what is designated as "good" and what "bad" is a site of constant social struggle and exchange, implicating bodies that are not just physical but classed, sexed, raced, habitual, historical. Our cultural choices mark and identify us. By developing them, arguing over them, and refining them, we are locating ourselves socially and identifying and differentiating ourselves in relation to others. In this sense, exchanges over value are never only about "likes and dislikes as such, but about ways of listening, about ways of hearing, about ways of being."[38]

Frith's account of the field of music gives a sense of the embodied character of cultural discrimination. The analogy with drugs is apt—and often the relation is much closer than analogy. To Frith's football team backs and soap plots, we could add last weekend's ecstasy. Or tomorrow night's bottle of red. Take Robert Reynolds's account of the Mardi Gras dance floor:

> Anthony sidles over on the dance floor and asks "How are you sailing?" . . . A variant of this exchange is repeated throughout the night with friends and strangers. Enquiring after drugs, sometimes literally so as one's supply dwindles, is the common language of dance parties. It begins and concludes conversations, snatched amid the din of dance music. Drugs fuel the party—they are the night's currency of pleasure. "There's a lot of love in here," bellows the Black American, Diva, into her microphone, startled by the rapturous response to her first show. "Yes," I say to myself, my cynicism not yet suspended, "and a lot of chemicals."[39]

In his account of Australian rock culture, Clinton Walker similarly speaks of how different music scenes presume particular bodily states: "Psychedelia—acid rock—sounds like, well, acid. Australian pub rock sounds like beer, plus maybe a line of speed and/or a couple of cones. Reggae sounds like da 'erb. Disco was the sound of amyl nitrate, or 'poppers.' Punk sounds like speed, as did the first wave of fifties rock'n'roll and early 'beat' music. Stadium rock—INXS in the eighties—was the sound of cocaine. The Velvet Underground and John Coltrane were the sound of smack."[40] Though cavalier, Walker's account avoids a sense of bodily impassivity. He recounts how "in the eighties music split into two distinct, opposing factions, Mainstream and Alternative, both with their attendant set of stereotypes: Mainstream equated with America and cocaine, while Alternative equated with England and heroin."[41] In other words, drug choices take place within a whole world of meaning and cultural value. It would be a mistake, I think, to read this differentiation in cultural habits purely in terms of a difference in economic or social capital (though certainly these factors are significant). This would miss the power and meaning, among participants, of labels like *commercial* or *grunge* in the field of cultural value. Similarly, nondescript concepts like "reducing inhibition" are insufficient for understanding what is going on here, as the qualitative differences in these music scenes make clear.[42] These tendencies, including choices of chemical modification, entail processes of cultural classification and discrimination. They are ingrained in the body as habit, such that they feel deeply visceral and compelling. But they link also to sentient mythologies of taste, performance, affect, mood, and sociability.

It is also the case that a concern for the body—its safety and its limits— can play a part in these processes of cultural preference and distinction. Robert Reynolds gives a sense of this in his account of the activities leading up to the Mardi Gras party: "I love this part of the evening. . . . You gather with friends, divide up the drugs, compare booties and pill dropping schedules, and ease into the night with prickles of anticipation. . . . It's hard not to feel the frisson of risk, deliciously illicit yet carefully managed."[43] Here care is part of a pleasurable social activity involving habitual acts of planning and comparison that become second nature to participants. In their ethnographic study of drug use among Sydney gay men, Erica Southgate and Max Hopwood document the existence of what they call a "folk pharmacology" that informs safe drug practice in this setting. This is "manifested in judgements, decisions, and practices" that define and delineate what types of illicit drug use are considered desirable and acceptable, and what not, and includes considerations of drug effects, routes of administration, and the risks and harms of different forms of use.[44] Notions of competent drug use were embedded within the "mastery of a multitude of practices that make up 'partying' "—practices that include "choosing and wearing the right clothes; developing and displaying your body in a particular manner ('attitude'); dancing according to a certain style; 'cruising' for sex using a variety of understood bodily codes; and taking specific types of drugs and combinations of these drugs according to a number of folk rules designed to minimise the risk of one becoming a 'messy queen.' "[45] Being messy meant being "out of control" on drugs, and the authors list a number of practices and procedures intended to prevent this possibility. These include considerations of drug selection, timing, and environment, as well as measures taken around the anticipation of particular physical or emotional states. "Becoming messy meant ruining the pleasure of a good night out not only for oneself, but for friends and lovers. It also meant the potential forfeiting of a rather substantial investment made in terms of the purchase of costume, tickets, and drugs."[46] In other words, considerations of care and safety are often inextricable from the field of value that surrounds the drug experience. The authors identify a hierarchy of value operating within this field involving distinctions between, for example, competent versus "messy" use, different routes of administration, and of course "good drugs" (in this sample ecstasy, speed, GHB) and "bad drugs" (heroin, alcohol). Obviously, such distinctions and forms of cultural discrimination are not without their problems.[47] For example, the authors describe how value judgments surrounding some modes of use (injecting) served to dissuade participants from that activity, but also had the potential to socially isolate users of that mode. We can nonetheless see that drugs are linked to *specific* practices of pleasure and forms of sociability. They are used to produce particular contexts of interaction, pleasure, and activity. This entails a host of tiny routines and decisions about method, context, disposition, and desire. And these decisions are linked to a series of moral judgments around desirable sensations, uses, outcomes, and behavior. As Simon Frith says of cultural judgments generally, the concern being exercised here is not simply about the intrinsic properties of the object (the drug) or "what it means," but is also a question of "what can I do with it; and what I can do with it is what it means—interpretation is a matter of argument, of understanding wrought from social activity."[48] Most importantly, we can see that specific practices of care and attention are being brought to the question of how to use drugs, such that considerations of safety appear as part of a concern to *maximize* pleasure, rather than standing in direct opposition to it.

It is precisely this sense of care as a potentiality in the body that many HIV and harm-reduction initiatives have sought to actualize. Recognizing the situated nature of the most serious harms, they aim to identify and enhance the processes through which people look after themselves.[49] This creates an emphasis on technique, proposing a differentiation in the field of "uses" that is neatly summed up by the saying "how to do more safely what you were going to do anyway." In practical terms, this has generally involved acting on the environments and situations in which specific risks are taken—for example, the provision of clean syringes, the creation of injecting rooms, or the regulation of sex venues so that they provide condoms and lubricant. But when it comes to a more explicit articulation of pleasure, these initiatives tend to be less forthcoming. Thus it is with some surprise that Pat O'Malley and Mariana Valverde note the absence of any discussion of pleasure in harm-reduction educational materials.[50] As they explain, harm reduction incorporates all drugs, licit and illicit, "into a single functional category, and seeks to manage them by "amorally" governing the risk and harms they generate." But while users and potential users are often provided with information to make "informed choices" about the risks of drug consumption, and different modes of drug use get classified, "any relationship between drug use and pleasure appears to be ignored."[51]

> Discourses of addiction and abuse are replaced by references to the "drug user" who is regarded as a consumer in the world of consumerism, quite capable of making rational choices and of discerning between advantageous and disadvantageous commodities and behaviour. . . . Compulsions—whether in the form of chemical compulsions, physical compulsions, social-environmental or cognitive and neural compulsions—thus not only vitiate freedom and the play of rationality,

but for that reason are associated with misery and pain rather than pleasure. *Liberal pleasure appears as intrinsically volitional, for one who has no control over desire could not perform the calculus that makes her free and rational.*[52] (original emphasis)

Thus, while an understanding of the body as habitual and habituated appears to underpin some of the physical interventions of harm reduction, such an understanding is less apparent in educational materials. As O'Malley and Valverde explain, "The more or less explicit model of the subject deployed in harm minimization is that of the rational choice actor who will perform the felicity calculus."[53] But as cultural theory has shown at length, pleasure—including the pleasures of consumption—is not intrinsically volitional. Our tastes and cultural choices—including our choices in the world of goods—*do not* spring from some unadulterated exercise of sovereign will. They are acquired, slowly and laboriously, in the day-to-day round of existence, socially shaped, ingrained in the body, and naturalized by power—such that my discovery of listening pleasure in Kylie Minogue will seem as natural and irresistible to me as my colleague's selection of Beethoven or Mahler. This does not mean that change or learning is impossible. (I may yet get my colleague to appreciate the finer points of Kylie Minogue.) But such change is slow, unexpected, and never available to complete control. It comes about through experimentation and differentiation and exposure (sometimes uncomfortable) to others. Crucially, it involves practices of discernment, differentiation, and responsiveness—and no one is left unaltered in the process.

Theories of taste and cultural value provide a promising frame for understanding contemporary practices of drug consumption, including safety. But rather than reinforcing a sense of the decisional subject of neoliberal discourses, these theories confound it. If drug consumption is analogous to consumption in general, its intelligent use would seem to necessitate more opportunities to consider and evaluate the qualities of pleasures, not less. By evacuating pleasure from the field of concern, these materials risk reproducing a sense of the body as a freely chosen fate.

Sensitive Material

HIV-prevention education that has sought to engage the characteristic pleasures of those at risk tends to work in a register that is at once technical and ethical. It is technical because it concerns itself with "how to" questions. And it is ethical because it recognizes that these questions are always embedded within a practical horizon of concerns that extends beyond a simple concern around infection to take on questions of "how to be in an environment and in relation to other people."[54] Two recent resources from HIV organizations in Australia provide good examples of this style of education: *When You're Hot You're Hot* and *HIV+ Gay Sex*. Both of these booklets address themselves to particular target audiences —potential users of sex-on-premises venues and HIV-positive gay men, respectively. They are distributed through select venues, and their content takes the form of a series of "how-to" tips: how to use sex venues and how to be sexual as an HIV-positive gay man. This is a familiar enough genre in popular culture—the stuff of infotainment—though the topics these resources deal with are far less likely to be so generally available.[55] Already we are beyond the comfort zone of a position that would insist that people generally should not have casual sex, and that HIV-positive people should not have sex at all. These materials are noteworthy because they highlight the fact that ethical codes and principles come into play even in situations that are constituted as "beyond the bounds" of normative morality. They evaluate well; this is not surprising, since they answer questions that people have been made afraid to ask in public. Both resources contain advice on condom use, risks of transmission, and so on. But they situate this advice within the world of concerns as it appears to these specifically situated subjects. So in *HIV+ Gay Sex*, we don't simply have "how to use a condom." We have information on how to maintain a fulfilling sex life, how to disclose your status in a way that feels safe, how to feel sexy when you're constituted as infectious, how to negotiate a relationship with a negative lover, and so on. In *When You're Hot*, we have how to find your way around a venue, how to cruise for sex, how to communicate your desires and limits without talking, how to socialize in this space, and so on. This is very practical, very technical advice. In a sense it is no different to handing out a condom at a dance party. But it is conducted in a more textured or readerly medium. It is sexually explicit advice. But on this note Cindy Patton has provided important clarification: "[Educators] need to do more than produce shocking cartoons and confrontational slogans. They must develop better means of mobilizing the practical logics of erotic survival that already exist in communities, learn how and when these evolve in relation to the range of texts that intrude into or circulate beyond their borders."[56]

These resources work by making what are perhaps, for some, *unthinkable* domains of activity available to thought and practical consideration. They can be understood as technologies of government—as well as of the self—in that they aim to make particular fields of experience thinkable in certain ways.[57] It would be naïve to claim these materials operate romantically outside the scope of power. They are based on distinct practices of inquiry and intervention, and they seek to shape conduct in certain directions. They produce subjects. At the same time, it seems necessary to insist that the sorts of subjects and choices that these resources support are not subjects or choices that normative morality can tolerate easily or even allow to exist (which may explain the restrictive conditions within which these resources circulate). These initiatives can be characterized as engaging their audiences at the level of embodied ethics (as distinct from morals). They direct themselves to particular scenes in which people are making themselves into subjects. Note that the moral principle around nontransmission of HIV is still there. But it has been converted into technical advice that knows and affirms the embodied worlds of the audience each resource anticipates. The producers of these resources have taken some time to find out about the cultural situations in which certain problems come to matter for people. And they have looked to these locations for the conditions and embodied solutions to these problems.[58]

Counterpublic Health

I now want to consider some of the conditions in which this genre of education operates.[59] And one of the things this genre of sensitive education keeps bumping up against is the abstract body of public address. The scenario is familiar. A workshop teaching gay men how to negotiate anal sex is picked up by a tabloid. The newspaper takes a punt that this will get a good run with its readers, who are presumed not to enjoy anal sex, and it goes into a mode of moral outrage. The story gets picked up by a shock jock and dominates talkback radio for a couple of hours. The minister's office panics and condemns the organization or resource. This is how public morality works. It is a constant possibility. And it is very damaging because it compromises the ability of educators to engage people at the level of their everyday embodied practice.

In calling this the abstract body of public address, I refer to the fact that this dynamic is very much a function of the mass media's mode of address, targeting an imaginary national family unit that is both white and heterosexual. Simon Watney argued memorably: "Moral panics do not speak to a 'silent majority' which is simply 'out there,' waiting to listen. Rather, they provide the raw materials, in the form of words and images, of those moral constituencies with which individual subjects are encouraged to identify their deepest interests and their very core of being."[60] So while this conception of the moral public is an utter fiction, in the sense that few readers actually experience their "core of being" in this way, it also constitutes a forceful reality which HIV educators contend with all the time. It is easy to forget just how much this sense of a public body structures the activities of HIV education. It affects questions of content, design, and distribution, limiting the extent to which agencies can address bodies in these more sensitive, practical ways. But it also takes the shape of a set of practical assumptions informing the day-to-day work of educators—shaping which educational possibilities seem feasible or realizable, and how. And this leads to a gradual, incremental desensitization of interventions, where the desire to achieve mass reach is accompanied by a concomitant numbing of the terms of representation. It is a frustrating situation for educators, because one of the initial advantages of AIDS councils, as John Ballard reminds us, was how they suspended this dynamic, allowing the state to take credit for the strength of the HIV response while being able to distance itself from any programs that aroused so-called public dissent.[61] And if this style of education is difficult to entextualize in the case of gay sex, it must be that much more formidable in the case of drug use, which, as I have argued throughout, increasingly marks the rallying point against which modern conceptions of the moral public constitute themselves.[62]

Michael Warner's work on publics and counterpublics provides a useful way of conceiving some of the conditions in which queer and corporeal health interventions take place. In particular, it helps to conceive how styles of embodiment depend on particular scenes for the circulation of discourse, which are considerably more complex and diffuse than some theories of moral panic allow. Not only has there been a considerable expansion of media forms and types of audience segmentation in the past fifty years, but media are also an essential part of cultures that understand themselves in an oppositional or subordinate relation to the "general public."[63] While this doesn't necessarily eliminate the impact of the offensives of mass morality, it does allow us to conceive some of the conditions in which alternative positions unfold. Publics and counterpublics are arenas of discursive circulation in which subjectivities are formed. But in the case of a counterpublic, this arena has a conflicted relation with the dominant public. Warner develops his understanding of counterpublics from Nancy Fraser's work on the feminist subaltern counterpublic, "with its variegated array of journals, bookstores, publishing companies, film and video distribution networks, lecture series, research centers, academic programs, conferences, conventions, festivals, and local meeting places."[64] Already it is tempting to draw parallels with the institutions of what is called the "gay community"—with its organized media, magazines, bookstores, publishing companies, video lounges, research centers, dance parties, conferences, conventions, bars, clubs, political groups, sex venues, Internet sites, phone lines, and service organizations. But counterpublics are distinguished from "community" in a number of important ways. They cannot close themselves off so easily from exposure to others. They are expansive, they are mediated, and they are oriented to strangers. They do not have such comforting recourse to the fiction of mutual recognition to sustain their sense of social collectivity, and their modes of feeling are learned, not innate. Another important attribute of counterpublics—which distinguishes Warner's conceptualization from Fraser's—is that they are not necessarily or always progressive (the example Warner gives is U.S. Christian fundamentalism). As Warner understands them, counterpublics are simply publics, with similar expansive tendencies, but which maintain some awareness of their subordinate status in relation to the dominant public: "Ordinary people are presumed not to want to be mistaken for the kind of person who would participate in this kind of talk or be present in this kind of scene." Counterpublics "try to supply different ways of imagining stranger sociability and its reflexivity." And these attempts are realized not just in the content of their texts, but through language, genre, medium, modes of address, and discourse pragmatics in general. Their discourse is "not merely a different or alternative idiom but one that in other contexts would be regarded with hostility or a sense of indecorousness."[65] And because they are expressive of expansive lifeworlds, their circulation beyond certain bounds is likely to meet intense resistance.

What I find particularly suggestive about Warner's thinking here is the way he relates publics to particular embodied styles. Dominant publics are said to have their own language ideology, based on the institutions of domestic intimacy, which elevate "what are understood to be the faculties of the private reader as the essential (rational-critical) faculties of man."[66] This allows some activities to count as public and others only as private or personal. Counterpublics are also said to operate on the basis of a language ideology, but they characterize the world in ways that are bound to disturb this sense of "the public." They propose different norms of embodied practice. Thus, in the case of queer culture, Warner remarks that a "culture is developing in which intimate relations and the sexual body can in fact be understood as projects for transformation among strangers."[67] This is the sort of approach that seems to me highly conducive to the sorts of concerns I have articulated in this chapter. From the outset, HIV prevention has necessitated public discourse on "private" practices in a manner that has not only challenged assumptions about what is acceptable in such discourse but has also unsettled notions of *how* public discourses circulate in the first place. The enrollment of various forms of performance and interaction (drag queens, sex shows, pornography, dance parties) in HIV educational initiatives generally has consistently challenged the notion of the private reader as an adequate model of how the relevant forms of learning take place (though the aforementioned booklets do adopt this form).[68] Meanwhile, the counterpublic sense of limited circulation describes very well the challenges of doing HIV preventive health promotion. Frequently educators (particularly those linked to state funding) must contend with the possibility of having to justify their activities to wider publics or manage the risk that their pedagogies will show up in unsympathetic contexts. Perhaps most usefully, counterpublic theory provides a way of approaching notions of social collectivity that is not naïve to their ideological dimensions, but which recognizes the importance of a horizon of collective practice for sustaining corporeal change. A sense of collective subjectivity, as embodied in the condom code, is perhaps the most palpable factor in the success of gay responses to AIDS.[69]

From Warner, I get a sense of publics as frames that project the lifeworlds of those situated within the terms of their address. They provide a horizon for collective action and exchange, but they always run the risk of doing a sort of violence to the particularity of the bodies they encounter (a characteristic that increases friction and change). The booklets discussed earlier also work by projecting a background of collective practice to the ethics they affirm. But precisely because they aim to engage the lifeworld of the typical reader, they cannot escape a moral ideology, with the possibility of exclusion that this entails.[70] The moral closure of counterpublics runs exactly the same risks as publics. This is why these initiatives require open-ended inquiry into the worlds and situations of those at risk. The production of subjectivities is a risky business—necessarily, and often productively, so. It requires an analysis of how bodies are mediated—and participative forms of evaluation. Most usefully, counterpublic theory conceives some of the broad conditions and obstacles to the sort of corporeal learning that has been so important in the field of HIV. At a time when these dimensions are systematically obscured, it provides a frame for the practice of pleasure-positive harm reduction. Perhaps a good name for the care practices and corporeal pedagogies that I have described, which abound in these less normative spaces, is *counterpublic health*.

Conclusion

The care practices and corporeal pedagogies outlined in this chapter exist in a tense relation with hegemonic prescriptions around corporeal practice, modes of consumption, and relations to medicine. This tension circumscribes and constrains the production and circulation of educational materials that are grounded in the embodied practices of endangered groups. As well as obstructing effective education, one effect of this tension is to sensationalize social deviance as risk. Practices that may actually be safe with respect to HIV transmission, for example—or which may emerge precisely as attempts to find workable ways of avoiding HIV transmission, or construct collective contexts for the elaboration of practical ethics grounded in existing embodied practice—become sensationalized on the basis of the deviation they represent from corporeal norms and materialize as thrilling instances of transgression. This is the danger of what I have described as "exemplary power." Exemplary power works by taking certain practices out of their concrete and relational contexts and blasting them into the abstract space of public address. In this zone, any deviation from normative prescriptions around corporeal practice appears as a case of pathology ("addiction") or else reckless intentionality and moral transgression ("abuse"). Apart from demonizing individuals, the danger of this exercise of power is twofold. First, it eroticizes transgression for its own sake. Second, it promotes both public and personal misrecognition of the possibilities of care that actually inhere in given bodily practices. Elsewhere I have discussed how the moral panic around "barebacking" has promoted wilful ignorance of the situational and relational contexts of sex without condoms, for example.[71] Normative constructions of responsibility work here to undercut the practical or embodied ethics that are being elaborated in these contexts, with the effect of spectacularizing them only as risk.

In order to characterize this tension between moralized norms and embodied ethics, I have drawn on Michael Warner's understanding of the relations of publics and counterpublics to propose the frame of "counterpublic health." Counterpublic health names the ideological resistance to the embodied pragmatics of care outlined here—the elaboration of which I believe is crucial in terms of enhancing the well-being and pleasure of subordinate and endangered populations, such as queers, women, and drug users. As a concept, it tries to get a handle on some of the dynamics that impede the formulation of practical strategies of care within such populations, highlighting the sense in which these dangers are a function, in part, of hegemonic norms. Counterpublic health is not counter "public health" as such; the term has been devised after consideration of the remarkably effective and innovative collective strategies of subordinate groups in terms of trying to ensure their own health and survival in the context of threats such as HIV/AIDS. Nor does counterpublic health seek to impose norms of health on subordinate bodies, nor assess the value of subcultures or countercultures in terms of their commitment to public health. Rather, it represents an attempt to grasp the sociopolitical conditions in which certain dangers materialize, in the interests of enhancing public health.

Finally, in foregrounding oppositional politics, "counterpublic health" could be misread as an investment in transgression for its own sake—though now in the name of public health. But it is precisely the ways in which certain, much more specific practices and experiences of the body get reified as transgression pure and simple—as though transgression were their only value—that "counterpublic health" contests. To interpret the sex and drug practices considered in this book as only about transgression and escape is an inattentive reading of the pleasures and possibilities of subordinated bodies. Certainly, when it comes to the well-being of such bodies, it is often necessary to transgress social prescriptions around what it is possible to say and do. These social prescriptions are loaded against the adoption of more careful and attentive postures toward the embodied experience of subjects thereby deemed illicit, as I have argued throughout. The tension is particularly acutely felt in the fields of HIV prevention and drug harm reduction today, where normalizing therapeutic discourses are consistently cited to block the development of practical sex and drug pedagogies that admit of, and seek to work with, pleasure. Indeed, the elaboration of "care of the self" and "bodies and pleasures" within critical health practice paradoxically involves a struggle *against* individualization, particularly the forms of privatization associated with the neoliberal state.[72] The social making of the "bad example" effectively sensationalizes social deviance as willful risk (or else compulsive pathology), in a move that produces unendurable blind spots, enforces blockages, and preempts more grounded possibilities of care. Given such circumstances, perhaps the most viable way to counter the unhealthy individualization effected by exemplary power is to move—as impersonally as possible—through it.

7

EXCEPTIONAL SEX

. . .

How Drugs Have Come to Mediate Sex
in Gay Discourse

A few years back, in a video lounge in Sydney, I had an encounter that haunts this book. I was approached by a good-looking guy, about twenty-five years old, quite straight-acting (whatever that means). We went into a room, and it didn't take long for me to realize that nothing sexy was actually going to happen. The guy was seriously out of it, on ecstasy I presumed. His eyes were rolling back in his head; he was fumbling and swooning. I was disappointed (he was quite a hot guy), but it would have been useless to continue. I indicated as much and asked him if he was all right; he pulled himself together, and we left the room. I'm not sure this response was sufficient. But he was capable of walking. And while I tried to reassure myself that I was not my brother's keeper—or his mother, for that matter—he was gone.

This encounter has stayed with me over the course of my inquiries into the relations between gay sex and drugs. It has forced me to question almost every claim I have made about the possibilities of corporeal responsibility at this scene. I feel implicated in this encounter. I feel implicated even though the guy was a complete stranger whom I am unlikely to ever see again. He may not even have been gay (or so I'd like to think!). What is my duty to this stranger? How do I enact it? The ethicopolitical tensions between autonomy and care loom large.[1] Another question haunts me: What makes this guy put himself in this situation? Why does he feel he has to *knock himself out* to be here?

Lest it seem as if I am about to launch into a familiar lament about drugs and the "youth of today"—that conventional and odious genre—let me say more about the nature of my response. Part of why I feel implicated in this situation is that I recognized myself in this guy. It made me think about my own use of intoxicating substances over the years (though, in this instance, I was as sober as a judge). And it made me think about the circumstances of my HIV infection, the diagnosis of which came as a complete surprise to me in 1996. I had regarded myself as a disciplined subject of safe-sex practice, almost piously so. I was in the habit of insisting on condoms for each and every sexual encounter involving anal sex; I prided myself on sticking to the rules. As far as drug use is concerned, experts might call me a "functional user," the sort of use that is typical in gay and recreational scenes. In my case, this involved the occasional use of drugs such as alcohol and ecstasy, which did not seem to interfere with ordinary responsibilities. I cannot recall an occasion where I didn't use condoms for casual sex; generally I felt in complete control. And through the fog of memory, a number of possible circumstances emerge which didn't involve alcohol or drugs. I cannot say that drug use led to my infection. But it's a tempting explanation, is it not? And since a question mark remains in my mind as to the circumstances of my infection, I couldn't help asking, "Is that what it was? Was I like that? Does that explain it?"

Before we all rush to fill in my blanks, let me say that I am quite OK with them, thanks. I can't imagine surviving in a space of pure intentionality, and I can't imagine anyone else surviving like that either. I want to keep this question about "what caused what" here open, while thinking about what the will to closure might be doing. And I want a different conception of corporeal agency, where drugs don't feature as such a thrilling and obvious escape route from the demands of normative intention.[2] What is at stake in answering such a question, supposing we could ever answer it definitively? Well, it might make me feel better about myself, for a start. Though substance use is not an approved activity, most of us have been intoxicated at some time in our lives—some more embarrassingly than others. I would be able to explain, both to myself and to others, what is difficult to explain without invoking a hostile and castigating response. We all know that drugs are powerful and bad. I could say that I wasn't myself. Then I would reclaim my strict hold on respectable intentionality, and maybe then I wouldn't have to worry so much about safe sex. It would help, of course, if I renounced intoxicating substances entirely. I might inspire others to do the same. I could spend my time worrying about intoxicated people and blaming them for . . . (fill in the social problem). Between you and me, I can't really see myself sustaining this behavior indefinitely. Maybe every now and then, just on special occasions, just a little bit of this. And maybe I will take these special occasions and little moments of exception as opportunities to do all those wonderful, naughty things that my moral self so rigorously suppresses. *Welcome to our world.*

It is tempting to think of drug use as an escape from an oppressive social order. And from a certain perspective, and in certain instances, it may be. But this perspective covers over the multiplicity of drug practices. And it denies the agency of drug users: the capacity of our bodies to be active producers of pleasure—and incidentally, care. Things like sex and drugs and other forms of everyday practice tend often to take place in a subintentional zone, which ranges between strict intention and unexpected accident. Zoning out, getting distracted, losing oneself in something, cutting loose, getting carried away, getting surprised (whether pleasantly or otherwise) are familiar parts of everyday life, and are variously valued. It's only occasionally that subjectivity feels fully determined by one extreme or the other—completely intentional or utterly prone to accident. Total predictability and utter chaos may be equally difficult to handle. On drugs (but not only on drugs) some incidents have the habit of verging toward the realm of accident, incidents which evade the scope of the intention. But they are not entirely accidental either, not in the sense that they are unavailable to insight and consideration. This quality is something many like about drugs and alcohol, and one of the reasons that people keep taking them in full knowledge of their dangers. The recognition of these moments of unpredictability can be one of their pleasures. With this in mind, this chapter can be viewed as an inquiry into the incidental subject—and the fluctuating conditions in which certain of its pleasures and dangers materialize. Drugs are taken for all sorts of reasons, from the mundane to the sublime. But if drugs *are* seen as an attempt to escape from a normative or hostile social order, what would it take to engage more fully with the texture of these escapes? What possibilities of care, what new pleasures, what ethics, what multiplicities might emerge?

Westernized subjects often turn to activities like sex and drugs—and music and art and eating and shopping and dancing and exercise and reading and grooming and socializing and Internet-browsing—precisely in order to lose themselves. The experience of losing oneself is part of their pleasure—sex and drugs perhaps especially so. But to date the discourses of HIV prevention and harm reduction have worked mainly to install a sovereign subject at the sites you might least expect to find one.[3] There are good reasons for this: for one, it is wrong to assume that sex and drugs are completely exceptional or entirely beyond the realm of care and attention. The remarkable histories of safe sex and moderated substance use prove this, while the contrary assumption is unhelpfully cited both to eliminate these strategies and to demonize sex and drugs and render them unspeakable. With this in mind, I want to consider the shortcomings of the doctrine of strict intentionality as a way of framing everyday practice, including sex and drugs. Recognizing how gradients of intention run through all manner of activity might even help to counter some of the ways in which drugs have come to participate in a moral drama of extremes, in which pure intention and total disinhibition materialize as the only available alternatives.

Part of this project involves critical engagement with the scientific, public health, and everyday discourses which make the use and effects of drugs more or less determined. In terms of self-care, there may even be certain value in keeping the effects of drugs from becoming—or being seen as—totally predictable. To return to the question posed earlier— *what makes this guy put himself in this situation?*—a number of sociological explanations have currency. In many of these, drug use by marginalized people is read as a reaction to social oppression—whether that of class, race, gender, poverty, or heterosexism.[4] In the case of sexual minorities, it is sometimes viewed as an attempt to quell the pain of social stigma or produce a zone of escape from the normative social order. From this perspective, one might argue that this guy can't even think clearly about his desires. He has to "knock himself out" to act on them. Or else drugs are depicted as a form of self-medication in the context of pervasive heterosexism—a symptom of, or reaction to, social pain, a palliation of the self in the context of impossible standards of performance.[5] This approach has the virtue of relating drug use to systemic conditions, in place of the psychologism that dominates the field. It may help to ground a more systemic response to the problem and promote a less punitive stance on drug use on the part of marginalized populations (which is more than welcome). But while I think this explanation is part of the picture and provides a critical backdrop, I am not entirely happy with it as a total account of drug use—even on the part of subordinated bodies. Drug use is confirmed as only ever a sign of some "deeper" or "larger" injury, while its presence merely confirms the group as one that is "defined and unified by suffering, physical vulnerability and powerlessness."[6] Where does this leave the agency of the user? Users' lives are defined solely in terms of deficit.

This might seem like an easy stance to take in the case of gay men, who are increasingly presumed—even in the critical and antiracist literature—to be entirely volitional, unfettered by context, free from constraint, middle-class, and white. But what is at stake in denying the agency of even the most impoverished and marginalized drug users? What is the effect of reading substance use—even "problematic" substance use—as always only confirmation of social victimhood? As kylie valentine and Suzanne Fraser have argued, it should be possible to register varying constraints on agency in contexts of social subordination while declining to assume that people's lives are entirely determined by the latter.[7] The binary distinction between "recreational" and "problematic" drug use, which is a feature of popular and expert discourses on drugs, reserves pleasure for the privileged, in a move that can retract any recognition of the capacity for pleasure and agency among subordinated bodies. The attribution of passive victimhood is often mustered to legitimize the authoritarian treatment of the socially disadvantaged. It has been used to justify increased scrutiny and authoritarian policing of already severely scrutinized and marginalized populations.[8] Moreover, in treating drug use as only and always a self-evident symptom of "larger" social injuries, the specificity of each is lost. Drug use becomes symptomatic of crude and reified social distinctions at the expense of a consideration of their specific cultural dynamics. The risks of relying on an easy distinction between recreational and problematic drug use are amply borne out in the recent experience of "party drugs." What has become apparent is that the properties of a given substance cannot be understood outside specific practices of use and consumption, which are socially modulated. As valentine and Fraser put the matter: "How far can we go with 'pleasurable' and 'problematic' before they cover over so many multiplicities that their utility is exhausted?"[9]

One of the reasons that drugs are such a difficult problem for community health is that there is no clear recourse to a politics of identity or sameness, but the tendency toward disidentification is also strong. Meanwhile official regimes of knowledge and governmental practice demand a strict split between subject and object which disallows more embodied forms of engagement.[10] Perhaps it's worth trying to dramatize briefly some of the problems with complete self-identification *and* complete disidentification as alternative responses to drugs. Returning to my friend, perhaps I have done him a bit of a disservice. Because haven't I been using him to talk all about me? Concerns around HIV transmission lurk around all discussions of gay men's substance use, but they're not necessarily applicable here. The guy may have felt bad in the morning, and probably lost his wallet—but in his state, he had a hard time undoing his fly.[11] That is to say, his "problem" is a little different from mine. To impose my problem directly here is to do him a certain violence. I may have recognized myself in this guy, but he could be anyone. We may inhabit similar social worlds, but I am not him. In fact, I may as well distance myself from him entirely, just to shore up credibility. It's not really my problem at all. The move is quite tempting, and not that hard really. I mean—he was *such a mess!* No, this analysis is not about me. And it is not about him. (Who else isn't it about?) To summarize, what is the problem with gay men's substance use, and how should "we" define it? I'm not sure I can give any answers. As much as I'd like to solve "the drug problem" once and for all, and devise a program of definitive action, these problems are a bit more intricate than that and may require something a little different to address them.[12]

The Problem Crystallized

Accounting for HIV infection—as well as what has come to be constructed as "risk-taking"—in the highly moralized climate that surrounds the fact of ongoing HIV transmission among gay men is no easy task. Gay men in Western centers are presumed to be largely educated about the risks of HIV infection and the activities through which it is most likely to occur (unprotected anal sex). While the latter activity has come to be constructed as "irrational" in this context, the desire for sex without condoms is actually not that hard to understand. After all, it feels quite nice. But despite the intelligibility of this practice, which is largely unacknowledged, the occasional engagement in activities known to put one at risk of contracting or transmitting HIV on the part of gay men is thought to demand extensive soul-searching and explanation, and this has given rise to a host of pathologizing and psychologizing discourses in recent years.[13] Notably, it is in the context of this will to knowledge that interest in, and concern about, substance use on the part of gay men has been growing exponentially, with crystal methamphetamine acting as a lightning rod.

Crystal methamphetamine is a powerful amphetamine that is smoked, snorted, bumped (snorted in its crystallized form in small amounts), and sometimes injected. Its increasing use has inspired increasing levels of concern and moral panic in gay centers in North America and Australia in recent years. It is the sexual risk-taking said to be caused by the drug, rather than HIV transmission through sharing needles, that has become the official focus of these concerns. The drug has been constructed as different from other "party drugs," dangerously addictive and a major source of new HIV infections. Increasing use of the drug has occurred alongside increasing rates of HIV risk practice and HIV infections in gay Western populations around the world, which have risen incrementally since the introduction of HIV antiretroviral therapy in 1996. Notably, increases in risk practice and new HIV infections have also occurred on the same scale in gay centers such as London, where use of crystal among gay men is minimal. On the basis of the imputed connection between crystal use and HIV transmission, some U.S. experts describe the situation as a "double epidemic."[14] An unprecedented degree of community investment in antidrug moralism has been the result.

Crystal began to attract a particular sort of attention when groups of anticrystal activists, many of whom declared themselves to be ex-users, began to organize around the issue in a number of locations. Criticizing the slow pace of government and the perceived lack of focus within established HIV community organizations, they cobbled together alliances and began running graphic poster campaigns and community discussions (see figures 7–11).[15] The central motif of these discussions, which is also reflected in the campaigns, consists of personal stories that recount escalating use of the drug for sexual purposes, culminating in HIV infection. Groups such as the Crystal Meth Working Group in New York and Community Action Against Meth Amphetamine in Sydney have created detailed websites,[16] and have formed international networks that

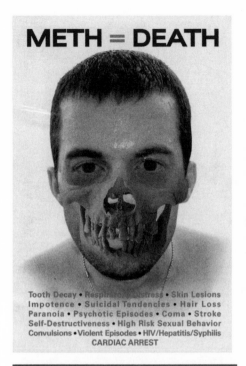

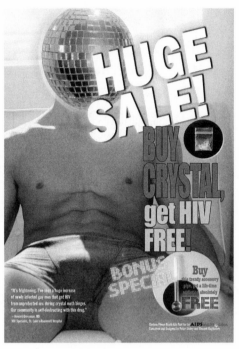

CRYSTAL METH IS NOT AN ANSWER

YOU MUST KNOW THAT BY NOW. I KNOW MANY PEOPLE ARE LOOKING FOR ANSWERS. PERHAPS THAT IS WHY MANY OF YOU ARE READING THIS. YOU WANT ANSWERS? WE'RE LIVING IN PIGSHIT. IT'S UP TO EACH ONE OF US TO FIGURE OUT HOW TO GET OUT OF IT. YOU WANT TO KILL YOURSELF? GO KILL YOURSELF. I'M SORRY, IT TAKES HARD WORK TO BEHAVE LIKE AN ADULT. IT TAKES DISCIPLINE. YOU WANT IT TO BE SIMPLE, AND IT RARELY IS, BUT THIS TIME IT IS ... HERE'S THE ANSWER: GROW UP. BEHAVE RESPONSIBLY. FIGHT FOR YOUR RIGHTS. IT TAKES COURAGE TO LIVE. ARE YOU LIVING? DO YOU THINK CRYSTAL MAKES YOU ALIVE? METH IS AS ADDICTIVE AS CRACK, AND MORE TOXIC THAN HEROIN. I DON'T WANT TO HEAR EACH WEEK HOW MANY OF YOU ARE GETTING HOOKED ON METH. TAKE CARE OF YOURSELVES. ALREADY HOOKED? GET HELP! LOVE EACH OTHER. THESE ARE THE ANSWERS. WE CANNOT CONTINUE TO ALLOW OURSELVES TO LIVE LIKE THIS! FOR HELP CALL 1-800-LIFENET OR 311

Fig. 7. Poster of the United Foundation for AIDS in Miami, distributed in Miami and New York in 2004

Fig. 8. Poster by Peter Staley, 2004, displayed widely in Chelsea, New York

Fig. 9. Poster of the Crystal Meth Working Group in New York, 2004

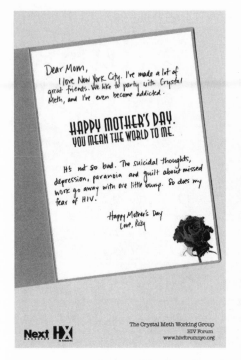
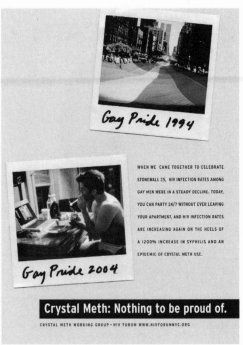

Fig. 10. Poster of the Crystal Meth Working Group in New York, 2004
Fig. 11. Poster of the Crystal Meth Working Group in New York, 2004

are generally critical of harm-reduction approaches and enthusiastically endorse the hard-line stance of conservative voices in government.

The fatalism implicit in the narrative of addiction does not tally with the experience of many gay men familiar with crystal, for whom limiting use to quite specific occasions remains somewhat effective in preventing the more serious physical and material problems associated with chronic use.[17] Nevertheless, the participation of this drug in problems not usually associated with party drugs—such as relational breakdown, social isolation, unbreakable habits, loss of employment, financial issues, eviction, homelessness, incarceration, violence, and the many very serious physiological and neurological effects of chronic or heavy use—has become a familiar story in urban gay networks, prompting considerable concern and understandable alarm about a problem whose shape is underdescribed by, and materially exceeds, the disciplinary commitments of HIV prevention. That is to say, the problematization of the drug within

HIV prevention discourse does not entirely capture the shape of em-bodied concerns around this drug, and this mismatch has been the source of heated community debate. As an upshot of this, a narrative of inevitable addiction is usually deployed by drug prevention activists in order to discourage use of the drug. While promoting caution may be important—and may serve to deter some people from use—this strategy does not acknowledge the practical experience of many occasional users of the drug, including long-term users who may have found practical ways to moderate their use, but who are generally shamed from the terms of the debate, or otherwise disinclined to participate.

Methamphetamine has been variously used in recent history, both clinically and within different social groups, to different effects—among truck drivers to clock up hours, among students to cram for exams, among street kids to stay alert and awake on the street, among adoles-cent girls to lose weight, within medicine to treat depression. It is in fact a common ingredient in ecstasy pills. Bumping became common in the 1990s on the sexually charged dance floors of the U.S. West Coast primarily as a means of enhancing stamina and mood. But the context of use becomes critical here. While the capacity of stimulants to enhance sexual pleasure was readily apparent to many participants in the gay dance-party culture of the 1990s, the instrumental use of drugs specifi-cally for sex has recently become a more prominent feature of gay dis-course in Australia and North America. Where the culture of ecstasy was popularly perceived to involve the dispersion of sexual energies to the more diffuse eroticism and communal affection of the dance floor, the use of crystal methamphetamine is now commonly associated with "sex binges," and, in particular, the use of the Internet to organize sexual encounters and private sex parties, where the drug is smoked intermit-tently through a glass pipe (see figure 11).[18] A minority of gay men now participate in two polarized and supposedly distinct moral worlds, the world of everyday responsibility and normative personhood, and a world of virtual freedom and escape, facilitated by the use of the Internet to organize sexual encounters and distinctive drug practices, by means of which normative prescriptions around sex, gender, and HIV infection are cast as less pertinent.

In neurobiology, addiction is understood in terms of the ability of certain drugs and activities to hijack the "reward pathways" that manage the normal distribution of pleasure in the brain, leading to a focus on increasingly narrow activities. But perhaps we need to transpose this terminology for the purposes of a critique of the highly polarized "reward pathways" of everyday life and their apparent inability to come to terms with queer pleasure.[19] This would involve a consideration of how the moral policing of public space contributes to the shape of this predicament. I want to suggest that the current manifestations of gay men's crystal use cannot be understood outside the highly moralized sexual climate of the HIV epidemic, nor the increasingly punitive forms of public moralism around drugs in general, and this drug in particular. Increasing HIV infections among gay men have prompted an increasingly conservative moral climate around sex, which has been bolstered by the intensely conservative political culture in the United States and Australia over the last decade.[20] In addition, there has been increased use of antidrug provisions to patrol gay recreational spaces and scenes around the world.[21] There is a growing literature on the ineffectiveness of such operations, in terms of how they produce more private, more dangerous practices of drug consumption as users attempt to avoid detection.[22] But these raids are only concretizations of a more generally moralized climate. It isn't the whole story, but it is worth considering the effect of such policing on the shape of using practice. In gay parlance, "do you party?" is no longer a question that refers to going out in public, but is generally uttered covertly online and means only one thing. As recreational practices get constructed as more and more unspeakable and illicit, they get drawn into increasingly narrow confines.

The Disciplinary Production of "Disinhibition"

The mechanism proposed for the drug-risk connection, in scientific and everyday discourse alike, is the concept of "disinhibition." This is the notion that substances can lead people with "good intentions" to engage in "bad behavior."[23] The substance is the agent here, by virtue of its biological effects on desire and cognition. "The impairment in judgment produced by substance use leads to unsafe sexual practices that increase risk for HIV transmission."[24] The concept is applied straightforwardly to substances that act quite differently on the neurochemical pathways— sedatives, stimulants, tranquilizers, nitrates, psychedelics. (Users of methamphetamine report a sharpening of focus, for example, which is quite different from the dissociative effects reported of ecstasy.) The concept of disinhibition is also carried over into psychosocial science to draw causal inferences from very general correlations. The reliance on simple correlations between substance use and HIV risk-taking for these purposes has been roundly critiqued within a considerable body of social scientific literature in this area, most of it published before the popularization of crystal among gay men.[25] Among those studies that do conduct the more rigorous sort of event-level and situational analyses called for within this literature, many find *no* significant relation between substance use and the likelihood of unprotected sex. In general, people who have unprotected sex when using substances are just as likely to have unprotected sex when not.[26] In the case of crystal, the drug's innate power to preclude condom use is presumed to be so self-evident that these methodological quibbles may be safely ignored. Yet one of the only studies published so far which has systematically compared gay men's sexual acts while high on methamphetamine, while high on other substances, and while sober, found no significant differences in the likelihood of unprotected sex across these different occasions.[27]

This finding would appear to cast doubt on the presumption of a direct causal relation between crystal use and unprotected sex. The drug becomes less available as an explanation for risk. Considering how drugs are invested in this discourse—precisely with the possibility of providing such an explanation—this throws a wrench in the works, leading experts to propose a host of psychologizing explanations for the "irrational risk-taking" that remains ("romantic obsession," "sexual compulsivity," "sensation-seeking," and so forth).[28] Perhaps this questioning of a causal relation is scientific sophistry? After all, if people tell us in qualitative studies and anecdotally that this is what the drug does, as is frequently the case, then why do we need pedantic statisticians to tell us what is "really" happening? Obviously drugs do something—otherwise one wouldn't spend such vast amounts of money on them! Yet what drugs "do" is an effect, in part, of the cultural narratives we have about drugs— narratives that are reproduced in scientific discourse.[29] In this sense, it really does *matter* how science represents this relation, for these representations substantiate an increasingly determined relation.

Disinhibition is a common enough notion, as mentioned, in everyday discourse. It conceives the social order in terms of a personalized moral drama between self-control and inner desires. But disinhibition does more than fuel cultural suspicions around intoxicating substances; it is also a source of value. Thus an ad for Hornitos tequila depicts an image of Dr. Jekyll and Mr. Hyde, suggesting that one of the things the product is *good for* is doing away with the constraints of everyday respectability and "unleashing the monster within" (see figure 12). In other words, disinhibition does not exactly "take people by surprise." It is a cultural script that is pharmacologically enacted. One of the striking things to have been uncovered in qualitative research is the strategic manner in which many gay men use crystal. Not unlike the use of certain therapeutic substances, gay men schedule their use of the drug strategically to enhance certain sexual occasions.[30] The drug is valued as being particularly good for what has come to be known as "uninhibited" sex. One man describes, "I use it for specific sexual encounters, if I know that there is gonna be certain activities involving anal sex that I might need to loosen up or be a lot less inhibited."[31] So while experts and anticrystal activists join hands to ascribe initial causality to the drug, gay users' accounts put this relation almost completely the other way round, and put the desire for "disinhibition" first.

Some sociologists have considered how the notion of disinhibition circulates in everyday discourse. They argue that, because drug and alcohol use is commonly presented as an excuse for "unacceptable behavior," it is necessary to treat such explanations with caution.[32] Being "out of it" on drugs may serve as a form of normative substantiation which attempts to mediate between bad behavior and good intentions. "Because they are commonly believed to be 'disinhibitive,'" Tim Rhodes writes, alcohol and stimulant drugs "may provide socially acceptable 'excuses' for engaging in sexual behaviours in which people may want to engage but perhaps know they should not."[33]

As mentioned previously, many anticrystal activists declare themselves to be ex-users and also HIV-positive. The central motif in their community discussions consists of stories that recount escalating use of the drug for sexual purposes, culminating in HIV infection.[34] Anticrystal activists were clearly motivated by a concern for how they saw this drug affecting their community. But there are also some grounds for thinking that this account of risk-taking and HIV infection could be operating in

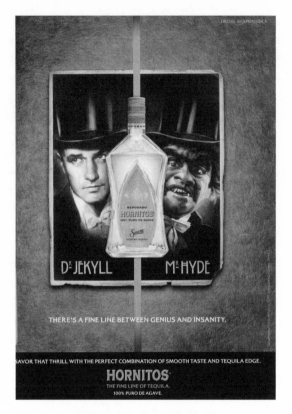

Fig. 12. Hornitos tequila advertisement,
GQ Magazine, November 2007

these spaces more generally as a form of "normative substantiation." This process works by constructing, as an innate property of a drug, a set of relations that are much more complex and may be alternatively framed.[35] As we have seen, this understanding of drug effects is not the exclusive province of anticrystal activists. It finds a wealth of support both in psychosocial discourse and everyday discourse. Its appeal as an explanation for risk-taking cannot be understood outside the normalizing pressures that compact sexual practice, HIV infection, and drug use into moral tales about the worth of individuals. Yet it does not account adequately for the materiality of pleasure, sex, and drugs, nor how these elements may converge within specific trajectories of danger—as well as precarious formulations of care.

Crystal is further associated with a range of sexual practices which, from certain normative standpoints, are considered highly shameful. Unprotected sex is one of these, but there are others. The drug is famous for turning masculine men—perhaps *especially masculine* men—into "instant bottoms."[36] It is associated with forms of sexual experimentation which fall outside the prescriptions of legitimate intimacy—sex with multiple partners, anonymous sex, so-called adventurous sex, HIV-positive sexual activity. It is used to explain sexual encounters that—how should I put this?—*pay less heed* to some of the sexual segregations surrounding age, class, race, body shape, conventional attractiveness, sexual setting, and relational context maintained by respectable propriety.[37] The transgression of imposing norms of personal respectability and sociosexual class implicit in these encounters is most forcefully attested in the testimonies of horror that frequently punctuate narratives of come-down, recovery, and moral restoration.[38] In the absence of HIV transmission, these forms of pleasurable interclass contact and sexual exploration might be cause for celebration.[39] But the prudent subject of drug discourse can disavow their pleasures and parcel them away as the scandalous effects of disinhibition.

By pinning responsibility on a substance, the discourse of disinhibition may produce that substance as a manifest form of freedom and escape from what are experienced as overbearing normative standards. The avenue that "disinhibition" provides for mediating between "good intentions" and "illicit desires" may make drugs seem like an essential mediator of sex in some circumstances. This would be consistent with the argument of some social psychologists that "for many people sexual risk does not stem from a lack of community norms or personal standards, but from a desire to escape cognitive awareness of very rigorous norms and standards."[40] They argue that drug use facilitates a process of cognitive disengagement from such norms which allows people to act upon their desires. The use of the drug for "sex binges" suggests an unsustainable tension between normative standards and sexual needs.[41] The availability of the concept of disinhibition, not simply to explain, but also to excuse certain sexual pleasures, could conceivably heighten the appeal of substances like crystal and make them more compelling. It could even be argued that drugs are taking on the explanatory role of the "unconscious" in scientific and everyday regimes that only seem capable of comprehending the rational-choice actor. Some gay men report that they *can only* have sex on the drug.[42] This is not a universal experience, and it might also be seen as a statement of preference, but the statement is striking for how it suggests a highly determined, apparently compulsory relation between sex and drugs. Can we just say no to this predicament? Is this sort of advice even practicable? I would argue instead that it necessitates a series of urgent sociopolitical questions. What are the conditions in which a small but significant group of people can *only* have the sort of sex they want on drugs? How do we account for a historical situation in which some people *feel compelled* to alter their consciousness chemically to even consider having sex? Given the increasing use of more potent and dangerous drugs for queer sex, could these isolated experiences be reflective of a much broader, tectonic compression in the moral landscape? What perversities of history and politics make the ordinary desire for sex and new intimate experiences so exceptional?

Uses, Pleasures, and Precarious Formulations of Care

Part of the project of "freeing up" relations between drugs, bodies, and subordinated sexual subjects might involve making room for greater recognition of the queerness that consists in sexual practice and everyday life more generally. I refer to those small "vacations from the will," mentioned at the outset of this chapter, which run through all manner of everyday practice.[43] Recognizing the perversities of everyday practice might help to counter some of the ways in which drugs have come to participate in such a moral drama of extremes. But recognition of the queer vagaries of pleasure must also take place in relation to the experience of drug use itself. For in fact my theory of "normative substantiation" does not go quite far enough. Escape does not even begin to describe the experience of drugs.

Indeed, by all accounts, sex on crystal *is* exceptional. The drug is said to maximize the pleasure and intensity of sexual encounters and enable experimentation and extended sessions. It is found to prolong the time until ejaculation and heighten other bodily sensations.[44] Not all users report a sexual response to the drug at first, which underscores the significance of a corresponding socialization process.[45] But use in sexual contexts is described as revelatory. The drug is said to give people the confidence to try things they might otherwise be too shy to ask for and to diminish feelings of awkwardness. "How to say this?" says one man, "What I find on crystal, I kind of enter into a special space. A particularly sexual, sensual space" in which "every touch is enhanced."[46] Given this erotic reputation, it may be surprising to learn that a common experience of the drug is the reduced ability to get an erection. But some men have found a remedy for this in the form of another recreational drug, Viagra.

The drug is also specifically valued in the context of HIV-positive experience. Crystal is said to make sex more conceivable and more enjoyable and give users the confidence to engage in sexual encounters.[47] Considering the phobia and social stigma that surrounds the very idea of the sexually active, HIV-positive individual, it is significant that some HIV-positive men see the drug as providing a temporary escape from the normative pressures of HIV-positive subjectivity.[48] The drug may be used to construct a different materiality, one less structured by concerns around HIV transmission. The assumption that sexual partners are aware of the risks and responsible for themselves is sometimes used to rationalize this context.[49] The practical difficulty of conceiving how to go about sex from this pressurized social location—and the virtual ban on peer-based, sex-positive, nonmoralized practical guidance about how to negotiate sex without condoms in a way that averts HIV transmission—may well make the drug seem like an appropriate alibi for having a sex life *at all*. The drug's reported capacity to enhance confidence, mood, and sexual sensations becomes all the more significant. Some HIV-positive people use the drug to deal with the negative affect associated with HIV diagnosis generally—which is not surprising, given that the drug has been used in clinical practice to treat depression.[50] In the context of the loss of friends and life-sustaining relations caused by the HIV epidemic, and the experience of loss and grief, some gay men have embraced the drug simply in order to be able to be close to others again, or as a way of participating in new, sex-positive social networks.[51] Other people just use it to get up in the morning. One HIV-positive participant in a qualitative study describes: "When I found out that I was HIV+, I didn't know what was going to happen. I didn't know what to expect with HIV. I didn't know where I was going. But after I started using [meth]—I started making some positive choices in my life. And actually I think I did some pretty good things. It helped me. I don't know how I would ever have got started again."[52]

ON THE ANTICRYSTAL WEBSITE of the Life or Meth Organization, Gary Leigh, the group's founder, gives an account of staying with a friend in New York, a friend he "had known for years as outgoing and exuberant," but who was now "just the latest of many to have withdrawn into the meth haze, contracting HIV in the process and restructuring his lifestyle exclusively around his musty, dimly-lit, black-draped apartment strewn with home-delivered fast food cartons, a sparkling new 17″ Mac to herald the arrival of 24/7 instant cable connection, assorted meth paraphernalia and a revolving door of Internet hook-ups of all shapes and sizes."[53] For Leigh this experience affords him "a sobering insight into a hitherto secret world," and his disgust plays a catapulting role in this account of his incipient activism. Leigh paints the "tweaker den" as the very embodiment of abject addiction. But I want to use this account as a way into considering further some of the microcultural dynamics of crystal use. For these subcultures have their own practical logics which deserve more generous forms of attention.

Tony Valenzuela describes a related scene in his remarkable account of the pleasures of crystal, where he describes "taking triple X-rated photos of myself to post online; requesting detached, anonymous role-playing scenes with multiple strangers; or seeking to be fucked unlimitedly . . . Often crystal made these experiences fervidly carnal in a way no other drug could."[54] Once you get past the intrigue that such accounts might provoke, you can see that this description shares certain features with Leigh's account—which suggest that this drug acquires meaning and value within distinct sociotechnical assemblages. It is no coincidence that the drug's popularity has grown in tandem with the movement of gay life online. With the stimulating effects experienced by users on focus and concentration, crystal would seem to be much better suited to Internet use than other drugs such as ecstasy, whose dissociative and disorienting effects I have depicted. What forms of online participation and webbed sociability do drug-sex practices involve? How do they wrestle with the personalization of the computer? Could the culture of private partying be approached as a specific socialization of this already pornographized and pharmaceuticalized medium?

The homes of some of the crystal freaks I've known and loved are "an organized mess" which do however share certain features: massive digital or video screens for watching porn, enlarged computer monitors and an impressive array of Internet technologies, drawn blinds, scattered and re-assembled objects, sports drinks, certain arrangements of furniture, specific sound technologies and other contraptions—a veritable orgy of multimedia. The drug's ability to facilitate repetitive activity and heightened perception is sometimes said to make it conducive to tasks which involve intense concentration without other interferences.[55] When not having sex, or hosting private parties, some chronic users busy themselves with private little projects, like maintaining their online profiles. Some houses are in a constant state of renovation. With the lights on, some crystal dens resemble nothing so much as your father's garage: total chaos, but it has a logic to it.

The appearance of Internet cruising sites has incidentally been accompanied by new online practices that attempt to negotiate sex without condoms relatively safely. The disclosure of HIV status—and the use of other, more ambiguous signifiers to this effect—has become institutionalized on many sites (not always unproblematically, but that's another story) and the practice of explicit HIV disclosure is increasing significantly. Private sex parties may involve groups whose HIV status is negotiated in advance, or regular couples, or solo individuals, and they may involve any number of sexual activities—both inventive and depraved—that pose little chance of HIV transmission. One of the more careful pieces of recent research found that substance use had no effect on unprotected sex among HIV-negative men, some effect on unprotected sex among casual partners of unknown serostatus, and some effect on unprotected sex among HIV-positive men. But the analysis also suggests that "with knowledge of a partner's HIV-negative status, HIV-positive men are able to enact their plans for safe sex, even if they use substances."[56] These findings would appear to bear out the idea that gay men use substances like crystal as part of an attempt to construct a different materiality, one less structured by concerns around HIV transmission. But they also indicate that, in the presence of well-articulated risks and practical strategies to avoid them, substance use does not lead inevitably to unprotected sex or so-called "irresponsibility." These strategies are not fail-safe, and require much better articulation and elaboration. But they might be approached as ethical techniques that emerge spontaneously within—or appropriate—new sociotechnical environments.[57]

In other words, unsafe sex does not exhaust the activities animated by crystal use—even in the most sexualized contexts. One hears reports of a range of disparate activities that take place while using the drug—such as chatting with friends for hours while smoking the drug at home; dancing; socializing; pottering around the house; fisting; fixing up things; cleaning obsessively; having wild, unprotected, piggy seroconcordant sex; watching DVDs; filming each other; browsing the Internet endlessly, comparing online applications, sites, and profiles; masturbating at length—whether alone, or with others.[58] Often the occasion is only nominally "all about sex." In short, HIV transmission is not an inevitable outcome of sexualized crystal use, nor does "sex" necessarily capture all of crystal's pleasures. In Cathy Reback's excellent study one man describes his "sex-binges" with one of his buddies as follows: He describes how he would be taking a shower or blow-drying his hair, when he would notice that his friend wasn't talking—and that he was, "like, in a closet." "I would assume getting something to wear. But you know—he would be in there tweaking—like finding all these things to put together. I used to say that his house was like the tweak museum. You go in and you see tweak projects and tweak towers and tweak jewelry and tweak furniture because it's all this stuff that has nothing in common with anything else that it is connected to, and it would form something that he apparently had a vision of at one time. Or just ended up with."[59] Different groups have used the drug in different ways throughout history, as mentioned earlier, and these have not all led to rampant unprotected sex. Club kids use crystal to go dancing. Some gay men use it for creative or work pursuits—before, during, after, or independent of sex. Street kids use it to stay awake on the streets at night and muster the courage to deal with prospective clients. One transgender participant in Reback's study claims that 99 percent of drag queens who inject crystal use it to "sketch on their face. They do their make-up, they tweak on their face." She describes a number of different activities that she engages in while on the drug. She uses it to walk, and to clean the house until it's spotless. And she describes "getting stuck." "Like I could get stuck in my bag, you know, stuck, for hours, in my bag—in my make-up bag. Just sitting, putting my make-up on. For hours. And keep on putting it on. And leaving it on. Taking it off. Putting it back on."[60]

These accounts—of "getting stuck," of getting lost in the closet—are what they are. They are funny. They are moving. They cannot be hero-ized. They are contingent. They are necessary. They just are.[61] They are nonredemptive instances of difference and repetition that illustrate the contingency of drug relations. When recognized as such, these moments of difference and repetition may have some practical value for those who are concerned to avoid HIV transmission. To notice these peripheral pleasures is to begin to refuse some of the more fixed determinations of crystal discourse—though such a refusal is difficult to sustain in the current onslaught of totalizing knowledge.

In terms of resisting "addiction," gay men adopt a number of strategies —though in the present climate these strategies are precarious. Ethno-graphic data is very slim on this, so here I draw also on personal observa-tion and speculative knowledge. Some users attempt to maintain a strict separation between their recreational activities (including sex) and their everyday sense of self. This constitutes a workable strategy for some, but one that may be compromised. For users who have jobs, the lack of sleep over the weekend and the physical effects of the drug produce tiredness and impaired concentration at work. In order to maintain their con-fidence and performance at work, some turn to the stimulating and focusing properties of the drug, and their previous containment strategy comes undone.[62]

For others, the disparity between their "recreational" practices and their "respectable" sense of self produces some dissonance, which can manifest in guilt, paranoia, and growing isolation. The schism between normative respectability and queer pleasure (Dr. Jekyll and Mr. Hyde) is relevant here. Some users divide their social networks into "respectable friends" and "weekend friends" (this is of course a response to the highly moralized public environment).[63] The binarization of social networks makes the illicit aspects of personal life difficult to reconcile with every-day social being, which in turn makes peer understanding, recognition, and support around these issues difficult to access in any safe or satisfac-tory way. Meanwhile, the continual presence of the Internet in everyday life as an instant form of distraction and virtual belonging, for both employed and unemployed individuals, works against the forms of compartmentalization that some gay men adopt to contain their drug use. The connection between online gay sociability and drug sex—virtually concealed but nonetheless persistent—makes for a particularly challenging if not inescapable environment to navigate. The decline in gay neighborhoods and their inability to live up to idealized expectations of "community" can make the actual experience of gay social life in urban centers seem bland and disappointing. The general monotony of working life and its failure to provide a satisfying context of queer belonging for most laborers lead to highly bifurcated and isolated subjectivities, in which leisure time is increasingly dominated by the need for sexual sociability—now rendered instrumentally as the pursuit of sex online.

For the unemployed and for those in part-time work or on a pension (many HIV-positive users), the division of social life into work time and leisure time is less available for moderating their use. In order to supplement their low income, some users take up small-time dealing— mainly to their friends—and the constant availability of drugs is not conducive to moderation. The possibility of a criminal record and the fear of employment-related drug testing hover around all these circumstances, threatening even more systematic exclusion from the workforce and public life.[64] Even in these severely reduced circumstances, many "crystal freaks" manage to construct a way of living whose small pleasures and modes of care, though covert, are not that unusual, but are rendered unintelligible and disgusting to the mainstream—an unintelligibility that compounds their bodies' disintegration.

Conclusion

In this book I have tried to suggest the value of an approach to drugs that is grounded in given formations of drug use and which involves queer practices of self-relation. Rather than insisting upon a sovereign subject at the site of drug use, this approach entails a degree of attention to and curiosity about *how the body is*, in a given situation—the queerness of its pleasures, their irreducibility to conventional predictions, scripts, and formulations.[65] This practical method turns to history, not to confirm that the body is subject to larger historical forces (which of course it also is) but as part of an attempt to multiply and "free up" possible relations among subjects, bodies, drugs, and erotic practices. It refuses to take current productions of "objective" knowledge as all-determining, though it takes them very seriously. And it does not rest simply on "having an experience," though it does take self-experience—and the claim to have it and make sense of it—as vitally important. Life may simply be more pleasurable and more possible when one tries to work out how different experiences are being produced. Biology is part of this production, but it is not all of it. Biologized subjects have other resources at their disposal. The archive of *using drugs* that is mainly yet to be assembled comprises a rich heteroglossic site in which the pleasures and capacities enabled by certain uses of drugs may be given original and joyful expression, and in which certain dangers are more specifically acknowledged. There are surprises and unanticipated experiences in these accounts which participants would seem to value or consider. Occasionally something new, unexpected, or queer emerges—a new sensation, an unusual mood, a previously inconceivable way of relating—and these experiences help some users devise parameters of use. Could greater curiosity about such moments form the basis of an ethical approach to drug use?

Given the negative physical effects of drugs such as crystal, some people will say that it is better to just say no to these contexts and possibilities. It would certainly be unwise to ignore the fact that, when used heavily or over a prolonged period, crystal is known to result in a range of serious physiological harms including muscle wasting, skin and organ deterioration, immune damage, tooth and gum decay, damage to blood vessels and neural cell endings, depression, paranoia, psychosis, heart attack, and stroke. As I write this sentence, I remind myself of the intoxicating genre of pharmaceutical advertising that now proliferates throughout U.S. media, whose lists of "side" effects hammered out quickly at the end must surely belie any confidence in the presumption of the inherent predictability of drugs (institutionalized, as it is, in the instrumental rationality of the randomized controlled trial) as they get longer and longer and funnier and more outrageous. But my suggestions here should not be taken to amount to a prescription for crystal, or for anything else. It is precisely against the medicalizing ideology of prescription that I have been arguing. In the context of dangerous substances like crystal, it would further seem that to discern any inkling of possibility in given practices of use is to run the risk of encouraging further use.[66] But figuring such possibilities remains important for those who are trapped in unbearably tight spots. I have been taking "use of the drug" as already given while seeking to refuse the normalization of any drug practice in this very intervention. In the case of gay uses of crystal in particular, the negative physical effects of the drug are typically used to ignite moral judgments about the sexual activities associated with it, which only adds fuel to escalating forms of sexual conservatism. The narratives of recovery that now saturate gay space conceive a pristine self engaged in "healthy" activities like sports, family, and "normal" intimacy. But this vision is depressing and, for many, difficult to sustain—and only raises the stakes of queer forms of experience. Hence the vital importance of clearing some space to account for pleasure consuming medicine. I believe a more open acknowledgement of pleasure and a respect for its importance in our lives is crucial if we want adequately to account for the social life and material effects of such drugs.

Practical ethics of drug use may be difficult collectively to elaborate within current regimes of knowledge, not least because they run up against the unspeakability of illicit drug use. Conspicuously absent from the crystal debate, for example, is the voice of the current user. The only authorized firsthand account of the experience of using the drug is framed by the discourse of recovery, the renunciative voice. Any attempt to question the self-evidence of addiction on the part of actual users is constituted as denial, their practices and ways of life as "condoning" drug use. For the subject of drug discourse, the unspeakability of their use within legitimate conversation would appear to consolidate "addiction" as a fait accompli. Users are bound to the mode of speech whose parameters of "true knowledge" are destined to fail them, rendering embodied or implicit practices of self-moderation virtually unrecognizable, practically speaking.[67] But while promoting more inclusive conversation is important, speech does not entirely categorize the scene of response I have been describing, nor does it completely execute the capacity for responsiveness—neither via complete inclusion nor preclusion.[68] Indeed, the speech of the well-intentioned subject can play out as a different matter altogether in practice! Given this indeterminacy, and the multiplicity of drug practices, it is probably worth jettisoning the binaries of moralized speech in this case altogether. In this chapter I have considered the inadequacies of presuming—and dangers of reproducing

—a clear-cut binary alternation between the intentional and the in-
stinctual or corporeal self when it comes to sex and drugs. It is also
relevant to consider that the notion of abrupt abandon—or the sense of
an unbridled and violent discharge of corporeal urgency from the scene
of ethical attention—only inexpertly characterizes the relational dimensions of drug-related activities such as dancing—among other cursory
scenes of imputed "disinhibition."[69]

Think of a dance floor. What we have here are much more incremental modulations of affect, mood, sensibility and subjectivity. Participants
are engaged with each other (or not) through embodied interaction and
an immense range of participative modes, diverse elements, and conditions. The various players are reading each other as they incorporate, try
out, come up with, and transform different gestures and responses in
various mixes of routine and spontaneous activity. A person or two may
be completely self-absorbed (possibly for quite a while) but that's OK.
They're probably working through something. Things can be boring and
predictable . . . for what seems like forever . . . and then they can pick up,
maybe through some small shift in the relational dynamic or some other
element—gradually and unexpectedly and increasingly ecstatically as
people get drawn out of themselves and into new relations and start to
embody new postures of attention. A rhythm kicks in. New things become possible. When a dance floor really "goes off," it has nothing much
to do with individuals, as any Party Animal will tell you. Everyone is
responsible.

Against the transcendent rationality that thinks it can work out once
and for all whether a given substance (or, by implication, its users) is
good or evil, or speak the truth of drugs as though finally, here I have
sought to adopt a more practical and "ethological" approach grounded in
given practices of drug use and their contexts.[70] The treacherous reduction of "the crystal problem" into "the thing that it is"—and the apparently determined enforcement of such conditions—make it clear that,
when it comes to addressing such issues, well-intentioned speech doesn't
always cut it. Resisting the categorical and individualizing force of "addiction" is a practice that does not take place in the pages of critical
theory or the health sciences mainly, but involves the critical and embodied work of consumers from all walks of life who elaborate their
resistance to bionormalization in varying but mainly hidden ways im-

plicitly and daily.[71] We are all junkies of one sort or another—or on the way to being made into them—though the differences between the embodied possibilities of resistance are irreducible. Just saying no to given forms of embodiment is, at any rate, not a collectively viable option. Given the problems that have crystallized, in the baser parts of this exercise I have been asking (and attempting to generate a more inhabitable climate for continuing to ask and answer openly and variously) the much more concrete, interesting, and not simply *urgent* but also *open* question: What, in a given encounter, is a drug-using body capable of?

NOTES

...

Preface

1 This quote is taken from an interview with Guardino that appears in Catherine Scott, dir., *Selling Sickness* (Ronin Films, 2004).

2 Ibid.

3 Preliminary analyses of the phenomenon of disease-mongering are collected in a special issue of PLOS *Medicine* (Moynihan and Henry, "Disease Mongering"). At issue for these critics is the "medicalization" of everyday problems previously regarded merely as troublesome inconveniences—a process that is said to naturalize certain solutions (the prescription of drugs) at the expense of others. They critique phenomena such as direct-to-consumer advertising of pharmaceuticals and the corporate sponsoring of research and medical activities, and point to a host of negative consequences of the pharmaceuticalization of health, ranging from rising health care costs to iatrogenic harm. But despite these important contributions, these critiques generally reinstate the professional authority of medicine in their efforts to determine "proper" diagnosis and the "rational" use of drugs, and fail to appreciate how diagnostic categories and medical authority always refer to, consolidate, and reproduce a wider field of normalization—even when properly maintained (perhaps especially). The idea that commercialization critique does not quite adequately describe, nor address, many of the important problems, is one of the themes of this book. I develop a slightly different approach to consumer subjectivity and subjectification.

4 Nikolas Rose, "The Politics of Life Itself."

5 More recently, the absence of pleasure from understandings of health behavior has been questioned. See Coveney and Bunton, "In Pursuit of the Study of Pleasure"; and O'Malley and Valverde, "Pleasure, Freedom and Drugs." See also the articles in the important edition of the *International Journal of Drug Policy* on harm reduction and pleasure (Treloar and Holt, "Pleasure and Drugs").

6 A useful sample of such work includes Martin, *Femininity Played Straight*; Cvetkovich, *An Archive of Feelings*; Halperin, "Homosexuality's Closet"; Sedgwick, *Touching Feeling*; and Elspeth Probyn, *Blush*.

7 Metzl, "If Direct-to-Consumer Advertisements Come to Europe."

8 The "cultural dope" first appears in Hall, "Notes on Deconstructing 'the Popular.'"

9 People seeking sex-reassignment surgery face a similar set of problems and compromising pressures in their negotiations with medical authority. The response by transsexual activists and within transgender studies is especially informative. See Stone, "The Empire Strikes Back."

10 Foucault, *The History of Sexuality, Volume 1*.

11 Foucault discusses the distinction in *The History of Sexuality, Volume 1*, 157. For useful discussions of the significance of this distinction for Foucault, see Halperin's *Saint Foucault* and *How to Do the History of Homosexuality*; and Davidson, "Foucault, Psychoanalysis and Pleasure."

12 See Rasmussen, "Making the First Anti-Depressant."

13 See Foucault's *The Use of Pleasure*; and *The Care of the Self*.

14 Here I have in mind Lauren Berlant's recent elaboration of the concept of "lateral agency." Berlant, "Slow Death."

15 The formulation "cultural dupe" appears just as frequently in the literature, but I've retained Hall's phrase to suggest a connection with popular constructions of drugs (see chapter 3). Pleasure is not a central focus of Birmingham cultural studies, but becomes nearly synonymous with the concept of resistance in subsequent literature that draws from this school.

1. Pleasure Consuming Medicine

1 K. Young, "Disembodiment."

2 See, for example, Merrilyn Walton, *The Cosmetic Surgery Report* (New South Wales: Health Care Complaints Commission, 1999). Interestingly, gender reassignment is classed in this report as a reconstructive rather than a cosmetic procedure.

3 This question inspires a growing amount of work in the sociology of science and medicine. A neat framing of it exists in Rose, "The Politics of Life Itself."

4 Kramer, *Listening to Prozac*, xvi.

5 Ibid., 247, 246.

6 Moynihan, "The Making of a Disease."

7 Ibid., 45.

8 I refer to the rapid response entries for this article on the BMJ website (http://www.bmj.com).

9   There are parallels here with the political strategies necessitated by identity politics. See Brown, *States of Injury*.

10 Shere Hite, "Try a Little Tenderness," *Sydney Morning Herald*, 27 January 2003.

11 Germaine Greer, "Viagra: A Soft Option?" *The Guardian*, 24 January 1999.

12 It is only *some* bodies that are routinely consigned to the sphere of "life-style," that are excluded from counting in any "necessary" or public way.

13 Mark Harrington, "'We Don't Need Another Venue': Meeting on Global Treatment Access, or Industry Sideshow?" (New York: Treatment Action Group, 2001), www.aidsinfonyc.org (accessed 14 June 2002).

14 See Rose, "The Politics of Life Itself," 15.

15 Trouiller et al., "Drug Development for Neglected Diseases."

16 Quoted in Britain, "On Drugs," 4.

17 Olmo, "The Hidden Face of Drugs," 10.

18 Daniel Kevles, "A Culture of Risk," *New York Times*, 25 May 1997.

19 Greer, "Viagra: A Soft Option?" In this instance, this move involves exploiting the cultural fears and misconceptions surrounding certain classes of its users: "teenagers of both sexes, aware that Viagra is a drug to be abused like any other, are following the trail blazed by gay men."

20 First reported in James, "Protease Inhibitors' Metabolic Side-Effects." In clinical discourse, lipodystrophy is now broken down into *lipodystrophy*, which comprises the former cluster of symptoms, and *lipoatrophy*, which comprises the latter wasting effects.

21 Kane Race et al., *Adherence and Communication: Reports from a Study of HIV General Practice* (National Centre in HIV Social Research, 2001).

22 Hardt and Negri, *Empire*, 92. They are referring to the "posthuman humanism" of the later volumes of Michel Foucault's *The History of Sexuality*.

23 There are inevitably risks in delivering up for collective determination the most nakedly vulnerable bodies, but these are precisely the risks the capitalist consumer context reproduces in new and more nonchalant forms.

24 Evans, *Sexual Citizenship*, 7. Evans's otherwise rigorous and incisive study is hampered by a tendency to construe sexual minorities as somehow more fully identified with the market than their heterosexual counterparts. This is a tendency I try to contest in this chapter. But in fact any familiarity with the intensive marketing aimed at new parents and their babies should be enough to disabuse anyone of this view.

25 Ross, *No Respect*, 203.

26 Paola Totaro, "Drug Campaign Not Hard Line Enough for P.M.," *Sydney Morning Herald*, 7 July 2000. The title was later modified to the slightly milder, *Our Strongest Defence Against the Drug Problem . . . Families*. I analyze this campaign in chapter 4.

27 Recent operations carried out as part of Thailand's War on Drugs and its Social and Moral Order campaign bear striking correspondences, for example. See Phongpaichit and Baker, *Thaksin*. The use of antidrug provisions to police queer social spaces is a feature of many recent operations in North America, but could also be considered continuous with the use of liquor licensing provisions throughout the twentieth century to do the same. See Chauncey, *Gay New York*.

28 Berlant, *The Queen of America Goes to Washington City*.

29 I am thinking of work that considers how heteronormativity naturalizes certain political economic arrangements. See for example Duggan, *The Twilight of Equality?*; Berlant, *The Queen of America Goes to Washington City*; Berlant and Warner, "Sex in Public"; Butler, "Merely Cultural"; Povinelli, *The Empire of Love*. I discuss how these forms of privatization play out in antidrug discourse in chapter 4.

30 Southgate and Hopwood, "The Role of Folk Pharmacology and Lay Experts in Harm Reduction." I discuss some of these practices in greater detail in chapter 6.

31 See chapters 6 and 7. See also Race, "The Use of Pleasure in Harm Reduction."

32 O'Malley and Mugford, "The Demand for Intoxicating Commodities."

33 In all the drug searches involving drug detection dogs carried out in NSW over a two-year review period, illicit drugs were found in only 26 percent of the searches conducted. Meanwhile, among the 10, 211 indications made by drug detection dogs, only 1.4 percent yielded "traffickable" quantities of drugs, and only 19 people were successfully prosecuted on this count in the two-year review period: 0.2 percent of all indications. In addition, the inquiry received "various reports suggesting that drug users were engaging in risky drug-taking strategies in an attempt to avoid detection. Such strategies included: the consumption of larger amounts of drugs at once instead of taking smaller amounts over a period of time; consuming drugs at home and then driving to entertainment venues; purchasing drugs from unknown sources at venues to avoid carrying drugs; and switching to potentially more harmful drugs such as GHB in the belief that these drugs are less likely to be detected by drug detection dogs." New South Wales Ombudsman, "Review of the Police Powers (Drug Detection Dogs) Act 2001" (2006).

34 I discuss how the moral climate produced by such enforcement practices plays into the current shape of gay uses of crystal methamphetamine in chapter 7.

35 Jano Gibson, "Dance Party Shut Down after Drug Crackdown," *Sydney Morning Herald*, 26 February 2007.

36 Agamben sees the exposure of bare life as an inbuilt component of sover-

eignty in the making of a biopolitical body. Agamben, *Homo Sacer*. But Agamben casts little light on why particular social and historical domains or activities become subject to states of abandonment. For my account of how drugs have come to feature for these purposes, see chapter 3 of the present volume.

37 Henderson and Petersen, *Consuming Health*.

38 Rose, *Inventing Our Selves*, 162.

39 Clarke, *New Times and Old Enemies*, 131. He references Friedman and Friedman, *The Tyranny of the Status Quo*.

40 Sedgwick, "Paranoid Reading and Reparative Reading," 19.

41 Morrison, *The Explanation for Everything*, 144.

42 For example Simon, "The Emergence of a Risk Society"; Rose, "The Politics of Life Itself."

43 An important and lucid history of the early governmental response to AIDS in Australia exists in Sendziuk, *Learning to Trust*. See also Ballard, "The Constitution of AIDS in Australia"; Bartos, "The Queer Excess of Public Health Policy."

44 Commonly referred to as the beginning of the modern gay rights movement in the United States, the Stonewall Riots involved a series of violent clashes between homosexuals and police in response to police harassment of gay bars in New York in 1969.

45 To give some sense of the scale of this event, at its height the parade saw crowds in excess of six hundred thousand people lining the Sydney city streets, while the main dance party had been known to attract over twenty thousand people to an event whose proximity to the parade made it more widely accessible and diverse than the regimented conditions of the North American circuit party might suggest. However, I don't think my analysis of the Mardi Gras dance party, which follows, is irrelevant to that context.

46 See Green, "Chem Friendly." Of course, substance use has been a feature of many of the urban places in which a gay sense of belonging and pleasure has been elaborated historically, including bars, discos, streets, and nightclubs. See for example Holleran, *Dancer from the Dance*; Chauncey, *Gay New York*; Ford and Tyler, *The Young and Evil*.

47 Delany, *The Motion of Light in Water*, 174.

48 Ibid.

49 Scott, "Experience," 34–35, quoting Karen Swann and Samuel Delany respectively.

50 In my view, the reference to the production of *affect* in the policy phrase "communities affected by HIV/AIDS" is a better formulation than notions of collectivity based on sexual identity or HIV status. The community I am referring to here was not delimited by sexuality or serostatus, but mate-

rialized through a set of affective responses to the epidemic and through the cultivation of different sensibilities. See further my discussion in chapter 5.

51 Sylvester/Wirrick, *You Make Me Feel (Mighty Real)* (Fantasy Records, 1978).

52 Gatens, *Imaginary Bodies*.

53 Saunders, *Ecstasy and the Dance Culture*, 36.

54 Michael Hurley raises the idea of "designer drugs" as "a primary inducer of tribal belonging" in gay and lesbian Sydney in Hurley, "Sydney." Further sociological analyses of the significance of drug use in this context include Lewis and Ross, *A Select Body*; Southgate and Hopwood, "Mardi Gras Says 'Be Drug Free.'" And internationally, Bardella, "Pilgrimages of the Plagued"; Westhaver, "Coming out of Your Skin"; Green, "Chem Friendly."

55 The AIDS educator Alan Brotherton has remarked on a time when it was not unusual to find "promote community attachment" listed as an objective in health intervention outlines. Alan Brotherton, paper presented at the HIV/AIDS, Hepatitis, and Related Diseases Social Research and Education conference, University of New South Wales, 17–19 May 2002.

56 David Menadue, "How I Got Tied up in Knots at Mardi Gras!" *Positive Living*, May–June 2002. The shared nature of Menadue's experience is suggested in one of the few other commentaries to acknowledge the effect of the AIDS crisis on the experience of the dance party: Geoff Honnor, "Looking for That Rush," *Sydney Star Observer*, 27 June 2002. Further support for the proposition that the "AIDS crisis" was a significant condition of the experience of the dance party can be found in Bardella, "Pilgrimages of the Plagued"; Lewis and Ross, *Select Body*.

57 Benjamin, "The Work of Art in the Age of Mechanical Reproduction," 222.

58 For a theorization of queer dance-party practice along these lines, see Bollen, "Sexing the Dance at Sleaze Ball 1994."

59 Honnor, "Looking for That Rush," *Sydney Star Observer*, 27 June 2002.

60 McGregor, *Chemical Palace*, 27–28.

61 For a critical discussion of such conceptions of community, see Iris Marion Young, *Justice and the Politics of Difference*, 226–36. For an alternative conception of community that lives in difference, see Diprose, "The Hand That Writes Community in Blood."

62 Benjamin, "The Work of Art in the Age of Mechanical Reproduction," 227–28.

63 Thornton, *Club Cultures*, 144.

64 Benjamin, "The Work of Art in the Age of Mechanical Reproduction," 233.

65 Again, by fabrication I don't mean that it was false, but that it was actively made through particular techniques and practices.

66 "We have to avoid nostalgia for what was and what has disappeared while creating a new formulation for future spaces and architectures." Delany, *Times Square Red, Times Square Blue*. But perhaps nostalgia has a more

critical part to play than Delany acknowledges, even in his own analysis. For a thought-provoking argument on the relation between nostalgia and sexual politics in neoconservative society that suggests that this is the case, see Castiglia, "Sex Panics, Sex Publics, Sex Memories."

67 See generally the final chapter of Halberstam, *In a Queer Time and Place.* Halberstam draws on the work of Jean-Luc Nancy to discuss the nostalgia of community.

68 On purification, see Latour, *We Have Never Been Modern.* The political romanticization of the natural and the organic is powerfully contested in Haraway, "A Cyborg Manifesto."

69 Keane, *What's Wrong with Addiction?*, 29.

70 I have in mind here Donna Haraway's notion of embodied vision. See Haraway, "Situated Knowledges."

2. Prescribing the Self

1 The passage from David Menadue quoted in chapter 1 offers evidence of this. He discusses how the introduction of HIV treatment combinations produced a different sense of the future for him, leaving him to ponder "supposedly normal things. Like: what am I doing sauntering around Mardi Gras dancefloors in my fiftieth year?"

2 Given the might of the United States in pharmaceutical regulation, bio-medical and evidential paradigms, and international drug policy, any analysis of the regulatory effects of drug discourses finds itself grappling with the predominance of U.S. imperialism and influence. Thus my analyses in the next few chapters can be read as enabled by, and attempting to mobilize, an alternate geohistorical positioning.

3 Foucault, *Use of Pleasure*, 11. For an influential sociological adaptation of this concept, see Rose, *Inventing Our Selves.*

4 Sackett and Haynes, *Compliance with Therapeutic Regimens*, 9.

5 Ibid., 1.

6 Ibid., xiii, note 2.

7 Armstrong, *The Political Anatomy of the Body.*

8 Haynes, Sackett, and Taylor, *Compliance in Health Care*, 4.

9 Ibid., 4. James Trostle notes this dramatic increase in an article that argues compliance is "an ideology that assumes and justifies physician authority." His target is the medical profession's view of its own centrality to health care. Trostle, "Medical Compliance as an Ideology," 1299.

10 Trostle, "Medical Compliance as an Ideology."

11 See for example Berridge and Edwards, *Opium and the People*; Temin, *Taking Your Medicine.*

12 Rose, *Inventing Our Selves*, 162.

13 Berridge and Edwards, *Opium and the People*, 49.

14 Peter Temin argues this latter point in Temin, *Taking Your Medicine*. A historical perspective less enamored of the free market can be found in Marks, "Revisiting the Origins of Compulsory Drug Prescriptions."

15 Rose, "Government, Authority and Expertise in Advanced Liberalism," 291.

16 Temin, *Taking Your Medicine*, 23–26.

17 Some bills and the U.S. model state law drafted at the beginning of the twentieth century attempted to limit the availability of opium, its derivatives, and other "habit-forming drugs" (including cocaine and chloryl hydrate) to doctors' prescriptions. These substances were subject to a different problematizing push by virtue of their association with particular social minorities. Early Australian opium laws betray this tendency, for example, by referring specifically to "opium-smoking." As Desmond Manderson notes, "the Chinese only smoked their opium and only the Chinese did so." Opium epitomized the moral difference and perceived threat that this new immigrant group was thought to pose to the white (immigrant) population. Manderson, "The Semiotics of the Title," 167. In North America, cocaine became the subject of legislative efforts when moral entrepreneurs rallied around the matter of its "overstimulating" effects on the African American underclass—though its use was common in various preparations throughout North American society. Musto, *The American Disease*. The temperance movement similarly reflects tensions between a predominantly Protestant rural middle class and a growing Catholic immigrant working class. One difficulty faced by these early crusaders was the fact that many of the substances targeted were staple elements of medical treatment: thus medical prescription initially constitutes an exception to prohibitionist efforts. The notion of "medical use" takes on a more determinative role in the designation of illicit drugs from the 1970s, as I discuss in chapter 3.

18 Temin, *Taking Your Medicine*, 47.

19 Quoted in Marks, "Revisiting the Origins of Compulsory Drug Prescriptions," 110.

20 Marks, ibid.

21 Temin, *Taking Your Medicine*, 47.

22 Interestingly, provision of consumer information reemerged as a key point of contest in the context of gendered disputes around the oral contraceptive pill. For women's health activists, the oral contraceptive pill articulated highly ambivalently with feminist concerns around reproductive health (especially in the wake of the thalidomide scandal), resistance to a masculinist medical establishment and its technological solutions (also perceived as masculinist), and support for women's sexual freedom and reproductive

autonomy, which the pill arguably promoted. A key achievement of women's health activists as an outcome of this controversy was getting the FDA to require detailed patient-information leaflets in the packaging of pharmaceutical products. In the context of gendered disputes around pharmaceutical technology and the rightful administration of bodies, the provision of consumer information was seen as a viable compromise that importantly intervened in the masculinist institutions of medical prescription. For an account of these struggles, see Watkins, *On the Pill*.

23 Armstrong, *Political Anatomy of the Body*, 104.

24 Ibid.

25 These 1935 studies are cited by Armstrong, ibid., 103–4. The "defaulting child" represents a concern for "congenitally syphilitic children whose mothers did not bring them regularly for treatment." Nabarro, "The Defaulting Child," 91. Armstrong also cites a "medico-social analysis of 381 women patients" from 1947 that attempts "to locate venereal disease defaulters from a social point of view." Though not discussed by Armstrong, the focus on (usually women's) wayward sexual behaviour is noteworthy.

26 Lerner, "From Careless Consumptives to Recalcitrant Patients," 1425.

27 Ibid.

28 A. D. Frazer, quoted in Armstrong, *Political Anatomy of the Body*, 103.

29 Brackenbury, quoted in Armstrong, ibid., 106.

30 Davis, "Physiologic, Psychological and Demographic Factors in Patient Compliance with Doctors' Orders."

31 Roth, Caron, and Bartholomew, "Measuring Intake of a Prescribed Medication," 236.

32 Ibid.

33 Ibid., 230.

34 Rosenstock, "Patients' Compliance with Health Regimens," 403.

35 Stimson, "Obeying Doctor's Orders."

36 Conrad, "The Meaning of Medications," 29; Amarasingham, "Social and Cultural Perspectives on Medication Refusal."

37 Conrad, "The Meaning of Medications," 29.

38 Amarasingham, "Social and Cultural Perspectives on Medication Refusal," 354.

39 Royal Pharmaceutical Society of Great Britain, *From Compliance to Concordance*, 12.

40 Ibid., 14.

41 Ibid., 12.

42 Balint, *The Doctor, His Patient and the Illness*, 1.

43 Ibid., 4,1.

44 Thomas Osborne, "Power and Persons," 552.

45 Ibid., 527.

46 Ibid., 526.

47 Ibid., 520. Interestingly, Osborne also shows how well this conception dovetails with the later emphasis on the economic aspects of general practice: audit, self-review, and financial responsibility. He cites the 1986 view of one of the proponents of quality assessment in general practice, that "Balint seminars . . . were in fact one of the earliest examples of critical audit in UK general practice" (529).

48 Armstrong, "Clinical Autonomy, Individual and Collective," 1772.

49 For an extended treatment of this argument in the context of sexuality, see "Sexuality and the Clinical Encounter" in Diprose, *Corporeal Generosity*.

50 Rosenstock, "Patients' Compliance with Health Regimens," 402.

51 Ibid., 403.

52 Ibid.

53 Browne and Freeling, *The Doctor-Patient Relationship*, 2.

54 Baron Lerner makes the connection between compliance and evidence-based medicine in Lerner, "Careless Consumptives."

55 Epstein, *Impure Science*, 196.

56 Armstrong, "Clinical Autonomy," 1772.

57 Ibid.

58 In the case of behavioral interventions, the controlled trial has been criticized for failing to treat individuals as social beings, embedded in history and culture. A message about condom use is likely to be understood quite differently in San Francisco than Beijing, or in 1910 compared to 2000, for example. The notions of randomization and control assume that pure access to a health intervention is possible, stripped of the confounding factors of social and historical specificity. This leads to a verification of interventions that work in these terms. For a succinct elaboration of these points in relation to sexual health interventions, see Kippax, "Sexual Health Interventions Are Unsuitable for Experimental Evaluation"; Kippax and Van de Ven, "An Epidemic of Orthodoxy?"

59 Sackett and Haynes, *Compliance with Therapeutic Regimens*.

60 An excellent history of how consumer activists have participated in this production of medical knowledge in the case of HIV/AIDS exists in Epstein, *Impure Science*.

61 Sevgi Aral and Thomas Peterman, quoted in Kippax, "Sexual Health Interventions Are Unsuitable for Experimental Evaluation," 17.

62 In the case of infectious diseases, for example, much more is invested in dosing practice than individual patients' health—particularly in the absence of effective prevention programs. And the threat of resistant strains of bacteria and virus caused by some practices of drug delivery remains an important concern.

63 In HIV discourse, the paternalistic imagery of compliance led to its replace-
    ment by a discourse of adherence, which conceived the issue as a matter of
    adhering to the dosing requirements of the medication itself, rather than of
    following doctor's orders, per se. In other words, the doctor all but dis-
    appeared in favor of a prescriptive relation between consumers, pharma-
    ceutical products, and health objectives, as defined by research scientists.
    But this is consistent with the thesis that compliance should be approached
    as a mode of normativity, rather than describing merely an oppressive
    relation of doctors to patients.

64 Publications arising from this research include Persson, Race, and Wake-
    ford, "HIV Health in Context"; Race, "Incorporating Clinical Authority";
    Race and Wakeford, "Dosing on Time"; Race, "The Undetectable Crisis."

65 Race, "Incorporating Clinical Authority," 84.

66 While the equation of viral load with "life itself" at this juncture produced a
    certain inevitability about this ordering of priorities, an emphasis on dif-
    ferent measures of disease progression (such as immune function) and the
    possibility of changing treatment, interrupting treatment, or postponing
    treatment, not to mention the production of better drugs, have emerged in
    the interim as viable clinical alternatives.

67 Rosengarten, "Consumer Activism in the Pharmacology of HIV."

68 Kane Race et al., *Pills in Practice: Approching the Patient's World in HIV
    General Practice* (Sydney: National Centre in HIV Social Research, 2001),
    28.

69 Pozniak, "Surrogacy in HIV-1 Clinical Trials."

70 This does not involve retreating from the materiality of knowledge claims
    or the systematic methods through which they are produced, but a critical
    engagement with them in terms of how they produce social reality. See
    Haraway, "Situated Knowledges."

3. Recreational States

1 Hall, "Reformism and the Legislation of Consent."

2 Ibid., 25.

3 See for example O'Malley and Mugford, "Moral Technology."

4 Episode 616, "My Future Self and Me," original air date: 4 December 2002,
    Comedy Central.

5 This conception resonates, I think, with that described in "Governing En-
    terprising Individuals," chapter 7 of Rose, *Inventing Our Selves*.

6 Himmelstein, "From Killer Weed to Drop-out Drug."

7 Ibid.

8 Idleness was however a theme in some early scientific reports—a term that

bears different, if proximate, connotations. See McCormack, "Marijuana Smoking Seen as Epidemic among the Idle."

9   I apply this approach to the problematization of gay men's use of crystal metamphetamine in chapter 7.

10 Isabelle Stengers and Olivier Ralet put it this way: "The one who controls is the one who determines how the technical problem will be posed and notably if and how it will take into account constraints determined by human values and interests. This determination of the problem is a question of political choice. . . . It is always possible to maintain that [a given] solution is a solution to a problem that is *technically badly formulated*, that is, to a problem posed according to certain *a priori* imperatives that have resulted in handing over control to certain experts and ignoring others" (original emphasis). Stengers and Ralet, "Drugs," 218–19.

11 A useful account of this period in the North American context can be found in Morgan, *Drugs in America*, 149–67.

12 Manderson, "Drug Legislation," 170.

13 Sedgwick, "Epidemics of the Will."

14 Manderson, "Drug Legislation."

15 My interest in the political articulation of the parent takes its cue from Lauren Berlant's brilliant analysis in *The Queen of America Goes to Washington City*. See, for example, chapter 2 of that work.

16 On the history of harm reduction and its relation to dominant paradigms of drug prohibition, see Levine, "Global Drug Prohibition."

17 See my discussion of compliance to HIV antiretroviral regimes in chapter 2.

18 William Connolly has observed the reification and conversion of generalized fears by means of antidrug discourse. See Connolly, "Drugs, the Nation, and Freelancing."

19 The Protestant lineage of addiction, first elaborated in early studies of alcohol, is well known. See Levine, "The Discovery of Addiction." With its intimation of immoral stimulation, illicit markets, border control, and a seductive imagery of protection, drugs have proved seriously attractive as a political theme in developing economies such as Thailand, for example, where they simultaneously propagate an intent to protect traditional ways of life, a barricaded image of national unity and security, an appeal to middle-class parental subjectivity, and the purported value of a personal ethic of enterprise and continence amenable to capitalist relations.

20 Hall, "Legislation of Consent," 1.

21 I draw this example from Dixon, *From Prohibition to Regulation*. See also Hall, "Legislation of Consent." O'Malley, "Containing Our Excitement: Commodity Culture and the Crisis of Discipline."

22 Dixon, *From Prohibition to Regulation*, 318.

23 The phrase is from Sedgwick, "Epidemics of the Will."

24 For example, Bell, *The Cultural Contradictions of Capitalism.*

25 O'Malley and Mugford, "Intoxicating Commodities," 57. Rather than chide modern culture, they put this association to work to render a usually abject practice intelligible and to make sane recommendations for drug policy.

26 Featherstone, *Consumer Culture and Postmodernism,* 59.

27 Cas Wouters, quoted in ibid.

28 Hall, "Legislation of Consent," 38.

29 See, for example, Wodak's lucid argument in "Taking Up Arms against a Sea of Drugs."

30 Crawford, "The Boundaries of the Self and the Unhealthy Other," 1347.

31 Ibid, 1353.

32 Pat O'Malley has argued that the utilization of more punitive techniques of crime control in neoliberal society should not be considered a throwback to older, harsher modes, but is entirely consistent with the normative instatement of the rational-choice actor. O'Malley, "Risk and Responsibility." On the persistence of "despotism" in forms of liberal governance, see Valverde, "'Despotism' and Ethical Liberal Governance." Scott McQuire describes the rise of a media-based "performative" self in which "the public projection of 'personality' assumes critical political overtones," in "From Glass Architecture to Big Brother." More generally, the political technology of exposure I am describing here resonates with Lauren Berlant's notion of the "intimate public sphere." Berlant, *The Queen of America Goes to Washington City.*

33 For a good analysis of drug testing as a mode of social control, see O'Malley and Mugford, "Moral Technology."

34 Hall, "Notes on Deconstructing 'the Popular,'" 232.

35 Clarke, *New Times,* 79.

36 Frith, *Performing Rites,* 13.

37 Hebdige, *Subculture.*

38 de Certeau, *The Practice of Everyday Life.*

39 Morse, "An Ontology of Everyday Distraction," 195.

40 Morris, "Banality in Cultural Studies."

41 Lawrence Alloway, quoted in Ross, *No Respect,* 148.

42 Indeed, it would appear that the hypodermic needle has had infinite symbolic use in terms of asserting a departure from established traditions of communications research. For a complicated account of the drug wars in this field, see Bineham, "A Historical Account of the Hypodermic Model in Mass Communication."

43 Even in Deleuzian cultural theory, the junkie body "seems to have emptied itself too fast, too definitively. Instead of disconnecting some of its organization and putting it to work in other reconnections, the empty Body without

Organs empties itself too quickly, disarrays itself too much, so that it closes in on itself, unable to transmit its intensities differently, stuck in repetition. It does not deny becoming, rather it establishes a line of flight that is unable to free the circulation of intensities, making other, further connections with other BwOs impossible." Grosz, *Volatile Bodies*, 171. The concept of desiring production bears parallels with the Certeauian notion of consumption as production, while the figuration of desire as productive and connective, rather than based in lack, may do roughly similar work in terms of steering "desiring production" away from given orders of subjection and toward productive connections—in a bid to resist the subjugating effects of capital.

44 Sedgwick, "Epidemics of the Will," 134.

45 "The Mass Public and the Mass Subject" (originally published 1989) in Warner, *Publics and Counterpublics*.

46 Frith, *Performing Rites*, 13.

47 John Frow describes how some strands of cultural studies suppose "a plurality of communities of value [constituting] the general field of value in such a way that . . . equality of representation becomes the governing political demand, and the subculture rather than the culture the meaningful point of reference. In some versions, now perhaps rather dated, this is a matter to be sorted out by the politics of contest over canonicity; in others it is left to the market in identities." Frow, "Cultural Studies and the Neoliberal Imagination."

48 Morse, "Everyday Distraction," 195.

49 Warner is careful to insist that the disturbance of identity is a "legacy of the bourgeois public sphere's founding logic" and *not* "a corruption introduced into the public sphere by its colonization through mass media." Warner, *Publics and Counterpublics*, 183.

50 Warner argues elsewhere that embodied identities can be performed in public in ways that are not about the representation of an inner self, but are nonetheless disruptive or transformative. Warner, "Liberalism and the Cultural Studies Imagination."

51 Gilroy, *The Black Atlantic*, 102.

52 Ibid.

53 Michel de Certeau, cited in Frow, *Cultural Studies and Cultural Value*, 49.

54 Manderson, "Drug Legislation," 171.

55 Hall and Jefferson, *Resistance through Rituals*. For an early exception, see the essays collected in Redhead, *Rave Off*. Today there is a growing body of work in club studies that references this tradition. See, for example, Sanders, *Drugs, Clubs and Young People*.

56 See, for example, Southgate and Hopwood, "Folk Pharmacology"; and

R. Sharp et al., *Ways of Using: Functional Injecting Drug Users Project* (Macquarie University Centre for Applied Social Research, 1991).

57 Morse, "Everyday Distraction," 193, 209.

58 Foucault, *Use of Pleasure*, 8.

4. Drugs and Domesticity

1 Foucault, "The Birth of Biopolitics."

2 Not be confused with "care of the self," as I explain in chapter 6.

3 Totaro, "Drug Campaign Not Hard Line Enough for P.M.," *Sydney Morning Herald*, 7 July 2008, 1.

4 Craig McGregor, "High Hopes," *Sydney Morning Herald*, 20 July 2002, 23, 30.

5 Paul Kelly, "When Johnny Comes Marching Home," *Weekend Australian*, 27 October 2001.

6 Anna Gibbs, "Contagious Feelings: Pauline Hanson and the Epidemiology of Affect."

7 My alternative name for this chapter is "Three Weeks on the Couch in October 2001," in reference to the period in which the federal opposition's non-attempts to formulate a progressive alternative to the neoconservative vision of John Howard's incumbent Liberal Party left many Australians glued to their TV sets in a state of left-wing despair. Of course, the defining context of the election was the September 11 attacks in New York, which saw Australia side with the United States in an inflammatory discourse of national security. This was underlined by a highly opportunistic election stunt in which Howard turned away a boat of Afghan asylum seekers to ramp up even further the national investment in border protection. Since they were typically seen to naturalize a demand for authoritarian styles of government and institute "security" as the dominant political rationality, these events are commonly believed to have changed the biopolitical landscape radically. But this chapter's analysis of the antics and imagery of the Australian National Drug Campaign—which was launched some time *before* the events of September 11, but strategically close to the election— indicates the preexistence of many of these techniques and rationalities in prior modes of neoliberal governance. Indeed, precisely the same social marketing formats and affective modalities as those used in the National Drug Campaign were adopted some months later in the federal government's antiterrorism campaign, including an admonitory TV campaign and a booklet mailed again to "every home in Australia," instructing readers to be "alert, not alarmed."

8 For example, *Traffic* (dir. Steven Soderbergh, 2000) found its way into local

political rhetoric. Not only does the televisual component of the National Drug Campaign lift some of its scenes directly, creating momentary flashes of visual and affective intertextuality, but also in his speech to the Inaugural Press Forum in 2001, the premier of the Australian state of New South Wales, Bob Carr, cited the popularity of *Traffic* as evidence, oddly enough, of a more enlightened, humane attitude toward drugs in the community. Odd, given that the abiding policy framework of harm minimization is on any measure a more liberal policy than the zero tolerance position promoted in the film (even the "soft" version that *Traffic* recommends). So the identity of the draconian past this example of humane progress is supposed to advance is difficult to figure. This moment encapsulated several defining features of contemporary Australian political culture: the nurturing of the press for state political projects; the poaching of American cultural forms to model "progress"; the effort to constitute an alert—if not alarmed—popular imaginary; and the currency of drugs for typifying the hopes, fears, and character of this constituency. Such moments efface local histories as much as they organize the future. They cite the discourse of progress in order to append political culture to a familiar set of figures—parents, families, police, and a putatively "familiar" Australia—employing the language not only of reform, but also of *liberal* reform, to import specific templates of domination.

9 Berlant, *The Queen of America Goes to Washington City*, 25.

10 Annie Cot has argued that the expansion of market logic made in the name of Chicago school economics into domains once considered non-economic (family and private space) invokes a fantasy figure whose function it is to reconcile love *and* money. The tender despot, as head of household, is invested with the task of satisfying the paternalistic nostalgia occasioned by the disintegration of the welfare state. As Cot argues, this fantasy permits an evasion of political responsibility for the social disorder caused by the restructuring of capital. Cot, "Neoconservative Economics, Utopia and Crisis." See the discussion in Morris, *Too Soon Too Late*, 183–85.

11 To expand slightly on the blurb of the DVD cover: Robert Wakefield, the new drug czar, struggles to divide his energies between the enormity of his office and his daughter Caroline's drug habit; Helena, the "trophy wife" of a wealthy but imprisoned drug dealer, confronts danger as she becomes involved in her husband's business in order to secure her family's future; a Mexican policeman, Javier, has his principles tested when he discovers the corruption of the general for whom he works; and, while attempting to protect a witness, undercover DEA cops Montel and Ray come up against the magnitude and seeming futility of their role in the "war on drugs."

12 "In the reactionary culture of imperiled privilege, the nation's value is figured not on behalf of an actually existing and laboring adult, but of a

future American, both incipient and pre-historical . . . not yet bruised by history: not yet caught up in the processes of secularization and sexualization; not yet caught in the confusing and exciting identity exchanges made possible by mass consumption and ethnic, racial, and sexual mixing; not yet tainted by money or war." Berlant, *The Queen of America Goes to Washington City*, 6.

13 One of *Traffic*'s most effective filmic devices is to conjoin diegetically discrete plots by joining them sequentially in one shot or thematic phrase. The effect of this is to emphasize the compression of (what are depicted as) radically incongruent worlds.

14 Connolly, "Drugs, the Nation, and Freelancing," 177.

15 Deleuze and Guattari, *A Thousand Plateaus*.

16 Patricia MacCormack, "Faciality," n.d., http://www.women.it/cyberarchive (accessed October 2002).

17 Deleuze and Guattari, *A Thousand Plateaus*, 178.

18 Ibid.

19 The suggestion is that this virtuously Northern cultural activity will reduce Mexican youths' chances of getting involved in the drug trade. In the final moments of the film, this specific form of hope and identification is again projected onto North America's poor Latin cousins: Javier watching a baseball game in Tijuana at night.

20 On the notion of racial-national capital and white aspiration, see Hage, *White Nation*.

21 Deleuze and Guattari, *A Thousand Plateaus*, 178.

22 Ibid., 176.

23 Ibid., 178.

24 The need for masculine authority is naturalized in the world of the film. Examples are Helena's competent but imperiled movement through the world of crime, and Barbara Wakefield's checkered campus past and implied incapability of controlling Caroline.

25 See Berlant, *The Queen of America Goes to Washington City*; Berlant and Warner, "Sex in Public."

26 Connolly, "Drugs, the Nation, and Freelancing," 184.

27 Quoted in Hage, *White Nation*, 223.

28 This took the (not uncommon) form of identifying the lived experience of economic hardship caused by neoliberal economic restructuring to the left-wing cultural and social reforms of previous governments. For astute analyses of this political culture, see Morris, *Too Soon Too Late*, 158–94, 219–34; Morris, "Please Explain?"; Hage, *White Nation*.

29 Mulvey, "Some Thoughts on Theories of Fetishism in the Context of Contemporary Culture," 7.

30   On the governmental investment in the family, see Donzelot, *The Policing of Families*.

31   Rundle, "The Opportunist," 41–42.

32   Ibid., 41.

33   The opening image of this ad, which shows a close-up of a young woman's face, upended, seems to have been lifted directly from the aforementioned Desdemonic scene in *Traffic*. The intimation of vulnerability and promise gone wayward seems to have been particularly poignant for both cultural imaginaries.

34   Questions of taste, embodiment, and class have been considered in Kipnis, "(Male) Desire and (Female) Disgust."

35   Tom Morton, "A.L.P. Must Pin Its Future on a Redistribution of Hope," *Sydney Morning Herald*, 26 November 2001.

36   Ibid.

37   Hage, "The Incredible Shrinking Society." This alignment is also evident in the aspiring goals of the bodiless voices: an English teacher, a mother, a fireman, a restaurant owner: a common language, a role for the parent, a state for emergency, and a place for small business: the key constituents of familiar ideologies of national unity and security.

38   Spigel, "Television in the Family Circle."

39   Lawrence Alloway, quoted in Ross, *No Respect*, 148.

40   Stuart Hall, *The Hard Road to Renewal*, 55.

41   Rundle, "The Opportunist," 42.

42   Ibid.

43   Berlant, *The Queen of America Goes to Washington City*, 76.

44   Tom Allard, "Labor's Stance on Illegal Drugs Will Cost Lives: Howard," *Sydney Morning Herald*, 29 October 2001.

45   Fia Cumming, "Women Will See Howard Home," *Sun Herald*, 4 November 2001. This story was accompanied by a feature in the Sunday magazine profiling Ms. Average: "Meet Ms Average: Size 14, 30 something, a mum, a worker, a wife . . . Politicians take note: this is the woman you need to win over." Maree Curtis, "Ms Average," *Sunday Magazine*, 4 November 2001.

46   Mike Seccombe, "Bowing out, with an Appeal for Unity," *Sydney Morning Herald*, 12 November 2001; Michelle Grattan, "One Last Plea from the Man Who Would Be Kim," *Sydney Morning Herald*, 8 November 2001; Tom Allard, "Suburbs Make a Fellow Feel at Home," *Sydney Morning Herald*, 12 November 2001; Kelly, "When Johnny Comes Marching Home."

47   Seccombe, "Bowing Out."

48   Deleuze and Guattari, *A Thousand Plateaus*, 168.

49   At the time of writing, families were being conscripted once more, this time at the other end of the *pharmakon*. With a New South Wales election

looming, their fragility was foregrounded with the hope of binding voters to the purportedly stable prospect of continued Labour rule. Once again, this campaign provided faces to latch on to, promising instant relief from the shared sense of alienation from the operations of postmodern government. An attractive young policewoman flashed across prime-time TV screens, arousing and absorbing nebulous fears, channeling their expression by presenting another cut-and-dried formula for virtuous citizen action: "People who deal in illicit drugs are destroying families. We've all got families we want to protect so please, help us get these dealers." An intense close-up mustered the reassuring intimacy and ostensible immediacy of face-time: "I've seen the damage these people cause, and I feel it's time to speak up." The missing segments of a suspect's dark identikit face materialized slowly on the screen, and I found myself wondering, where have I heard that compelling appeal to immediacy, conveyed in a tone of disenfranchised injury, before? On the affect of the televisual mediation of Pauline Hanson's face, see Gibbs, "Contagious Feelings."

50 A recent example can be found in Clive Hamilton, "Pornography's Unholy Alliance," *Sydney Morning Herald*, 26 May 2003.

51 This reading bears affinities with Heidegger's theorization of addiction, as discussed in Ronnell, *Crack Wars*.

52 Brendan Gleeson and Bill Randolph, *A New Vision for Western Sydney: Options for 21st Century Governance* (Urban Frontiers Program, University of Western Sydney, 2002). The analysis is Mark Latham's, who went on to succeed Beazley as the opposition leader for a brief period. Quoted in Anne Davies, "Latham Warns Labour to Hitch Itself to the New Outwardly Mobile Voter," *Sydney Morning Herald*, 19 March 2002.

53 Gleeson and Randolph, "Western Sydney," 21.

54 Ibid. By keeping the focus on the public investment of resources, the authors manage to avoid the cynical diagnosis of "white flight" offered by Latham, without neglecting how race features in the political administration of disadvantage.

55 Ibid., 25.

5. Consuming Compliance

1 Stryker and Whittle, *The Transgender Studies Reader*, 7.

2 See Gatens, *Imaginary Bodies*; Diprose, *The Bodies of Women*; Keane and Rosengarten, "On the Biology of Sexed Subjects"; Probyn, *Sexing the Self*.

3 See especially chapter 2 of Diprose, *Bodies of Women*.

4 On recent estimates, almost one third of PLWHA in Australia live in poverty. J. Grierson et al., *HIV Futures 3: Positive Australians on Services, Health and*

Well-Being (Melbourne: Australian Research Centre in Sex, Health, and Society, La Trobe University, 2002).

5 AIDS Treatment Project Australia, *A Different Kind of Roadmap: A Report on the AIDS Treatment Project Australia* (AIDS Treatment Project Australia, 2003), 20.

6 Ibid.

7 On counterpublics, see Warner, *Publics and Counterpublics.* I take a closer look at this work in chapter 6.

8 An earlier version of the argument presented in this section was published in Race, "Undetectable Crisis." Since I wrote that piece, the HIV response has become even more beholden to medical paradigms, sources of authority, and regimes of evidence, so I want to use this opportunity to identify and theorize what I believe to be some of the more interesting counterpractices.

9 Rofes, *Dry Bones Breathe*, 29, see especially chapter 2.

10 For a fuller account of this event, see Race, "Incorporating Clinical Authority."

11 Matryn Goddard, "Half in Love with Easeful Death," *Sydney Star Observer*, 8 May 1997.

12 Andrew Kirk, "Letter," *Talkabout* (NSW: PLWHA Inc., 1997).

13 Pozniak, "Surrogacy in HIV-1 Clinical Trials."

14 Juliet Richters et al., *Sydney Gay Community Surveillance Report, Update 1997* (National Centre in HIV Social Research, Macquarie University, 1997).

15 This analogy was made by John Coffin at the Vancouver conference.

16 Michael Flynn, "Compliance Ain't Easy," *Body Positive*, July 1997, 1.

17 Walt Senterfitt, "The Message from Vancouver: The Hope Is Real and the (Reality) Check Is in the Mail," *Aegis*, August 1996, www.aegis.com.

18 Marsha Rosengarten has analyzed the case of the anti-HIV drug Trizivir, which, though bearing the same side-effect profile as earlier compounds, is able to bill itself as a treatment advance on the basis that it simplifies dosing schedules and therefore purportedly maximizes the consumer's quality of life. Noting its failure to eliminate side effects, Rosengarten argues that this reproduces what she describes as "an unhappy split between what the individual subject may want from life and the requirements *of* his/her body." Rosengarten, "Consumer Activism in the Pharmacology of HIV," 104.

19 Incidentally, the increasing use of surrogate markers to evaluate a range of preventive treatments means this situation is likely to become increasingly common across a range of conditions. The American Association for Cancer Research has set the tone by calling for "pre-emptive strikes" on cancer in its formative stages and the recognition of a condition called "pre-cancer." Patients are put in the paradoxical (and, from the pharmaceutical company's perspective, lucrative) position of managing a "certain" threat using

inevitably uncertain, potent, chemical interventions. Preventive drug re-gimes produce a subject who is at once more consciously "at risk" of de-veloping a condition, and—to the profit of pharmaceutical companies—more impelled to manage this risk.

20 Law et al., "Estimating the Population Impact in Australia of Improved Antiviral Treatment for HIV Infection,"

21 Bartos and McDonald, "HIV as Identity, Experience or Career."

22 Duffin used this phrase in a number of HIV sector meetings in Sydney in 2001.

23 See Bartos and McDonald, "HIV as Identity, Experience or Career."

24 Goddard, "AIDS in Never-Never Land," 26.

25 The epidemiologist Tom Coates, quoted in Sabin Russell, "HIV Rate Surges: Alarming Incidence of New Infections Raises Fears of Scourge to Come," *San Francisco Chronicle*, 30 June 2000.

26 Morton, "A.L.P. Must Pin Its Future on a Redistribution of Hope," *Sydney Morning Herald*, 26 November 2001. See also chapter 4 of the present volume.

27 Laurie Garrett, "Eyeing an Ad Ban: Critics Say HIV Drugs' Claims Paint Too Rosy a Picture," *Newsday*, 13 March 2001.

28 The AIDS activist Jeff Getty, quoted in ibid.

29 Michael Hurley, *Strategic and Conceptual Issues for Community-Based HIV/AIDS Treatments Media* (Melbourne: Australian Research Centre in Sex, Health, and Society, La Trobe University, 2001).

30 Alan Brotherton, "Everyday Pleasures," *Positive Living*, July–August 2001.

31 Ibid., 2.

32 For a similar characterization, but one less specific to the HIV-positive experience, see Hurley, "Sydney."

33 Brad Johnston, "Got the Virus? Get the Lifestyle," *Sydney Star Observer*, 28 May 1998.

34 Ibid.

35 "Somewhere between AIDS activist and dead" is how another HIV-positive man put it in an interview. Bartos and McDonald, "HIV as Identity, Experience or Career."

36 Diprose, "The Hand That Writes Community in Blood."

37 I have adapted this idea from David Halperin, who makes an extended argu-ment for this method in relation to gay male cultural identifications in Hal-perin, "Homosexuality's Closet." See also, more recently, Halperin, *What Do Gay Men Want?*.

38 Race, "Undetectable Crisis," 183.

39 Hurley, "Community Treatments Media," 27.

40 Ibid.

41 Ibid., 7.

42 Thus, the camp rendition of the phrase "NOW! More choices than ever before!" has an ironic interface that intimates that "choices" are always made within particular parameters and contexts. It makes room for a critical posture on the idea that these choices are available equally to all.

43 Hurley, "Community Treatments Media," 21.

44 This point is increasingly pertinent in contexts where community organizations are restricted in their activities to the use of "proven interventions" (i.e., behavioral interventions that have been validated through randomized controlled evaluation), as is increasingly the case in the United States and around the world. This regime of evidence reduces the possibility of doing education that is grounded in the dynamics of local communities, or that uses more participative modes. In relation to the use of the controlled trial to assess behavioral interventions, Susan Kippax puts it bluntly: such conditions render "the interventions and/or the outcomes trivial." Kippax, "Sexual Health Interventions Are Unsuitable for Experimental Evaluation."

45 One only need consider the materializations of "side effects" or resistant virus (produced by the intervention) to realize the limitations of the sort of knowledge of agency proposed by the controlled trial. For example, some conditions caused by HIV drugs negate their therapeutic efficacy by making the conditions of their consumption intolerable. These conditions may be historically, culturally, psychologically, or physiologically contingent—or some combination of these dimensions.

46 Patton, *Fatal Advice*, 143.

47 Dyer, "Judy Garland and Gay Men."

48 Ross, *No Respect*.

49 See, for example, the discussion of drag figure Pauline Pantsdown, Simon Hunt's send-up of One Nation's Pauline Hanson, who has appeared in the Mardi Gras parade and been given considerable playtime on local airwaves, in Nicoll, *From Diggers to Drag Queens*.

50 Many Sydneysiders were shocked when a senior official at the Gay Games of 2002 walked out in disgust when a drag show was featured as part of the (locally directed) closing ceremony. Thankfully, this species of intolerance on the part of the normalized movement is much less prevalent in the Australian context—to date.

51 Leo Bersani has famously argued that "Parody is an erotic turn-off and all gay men know this." Bersani, "Is the Rectum a Grave?," 208.

52 Ross, *No Respect*.

53 Torres, "The Caped Crusader of Camp."

54 Flinn, "The Deaths of Camp," 436.

55 Ross, *No Respect*, 151.

56 Flinn, "The Deaths of Camp," 436.

57 Sontag, "Notes on 'Camp,'" 65.

58 Sedgwick, *Epistemology of the Closet*, 156.

59 Ibid.

60 Dowsett, *Practising Desire*, 70.

61 Bennett, "How Is It, Then, That We Still Remain Barbarians?"

62 Dowsett, *Practising Desire*, 70.

63 ATPA, *A Different Kind of Roadmap*.

64 These community forums are an initiative of the AIDS Treatment Project Australia (ATPA), a body formed in 1998 to conduct treatments education, consisting of people with HIV, community-based HIV treatment advocates, healthcare professionals working in HIV, and people experienced in health promotion. ATPA is supported by pharmaceutical industry grants matched dollar for dollar by the Commonwealth Department of Health.

65 Lizz Kopecny, "Kath Albury (Interview)," http://www.bi.org.au/culture/think/kathalbury.htm, accessed 14 January 2004.

66 For the purposes of HIV care, open discussion of patients' illicit drug use is necessary. Some antiretrovirals have severe interactions with a range of licit and illicit drugs (though pharmaceutical companies have historically refused to include specific information about the latter in their packaging).

67 Race et al., *Adherence and Communication: Reports from a Study of HIV General Practice* (National Centre in HIV Social Research, 2001).

68 Flinn, "The Deaths of Camp," 446.

69 While this alignment makes camp a source of concern for some feminists, who argue that camp derogates the female body, camp is better seen as a parodic take on the *conventions* of femininity and embodiment, thus enabling some critical leverage against the social enforcement of these conventions.

70 Ross, "Uses of Camp," 316.

71 Richard Dyer, "Judy Garland and Gay Men," 154.

72 Brad Johnston, "Lipodysphoria: A Growing Concern," *Sydney Star Observer*, 13 August 1998.

73 Cited in Flinn, "The Deaths of Camp," 436.

74 Gregory Palast, "Keep Taking Our Tablets (No One Else's)," *Observer*, 23 July 2000.

75 While embodied pleasures and political styles are specific to particular subcultures, they are not static, nor immured from one another. Consider how Mardi Gras and the Aboriginal counter-celebrations of the Bicentenary in Sydney (which commemorated the arrival of the first British settlers)

energized one another in 1988. For a discussion of how these events synergized each other, boosting Sydney's reputation as a party-giver to the world, see Michaels, "Carnivale in Oxford St."

6. Embodiments of Safety

1 Sedgwick, *Epistemology of the Closet*, 172.
2 Steve Dow, "Dancing with Death," *Age*, 4 October 2000.
3 In this article and elsewhere Dow links the use of recreational drugs to a culture of "barebacking" (a term that refers to the eroticized practice of sex without condoms in the context of HIV awareness) which he in turn links to the emergence of gay chat sites on the Internet. The association is not unique—Dow transposes U.S commentary on the phenomenon to the Australian context almost exactly. See Steve Dow, "Denial Becomes the New Language of Casual Sex," *Sydney Morning Herald*, 3 July 2003; G. Freeman, "Bug Chasers," *Rolling Stone*, 6 February 2003. For an extended analysis of this discourse, see Race, "Engaging in a Culture of Barebacking."
4 Ross, "Epilogue," 395.
5 Jock Young, "The Myth of the Drug Taker in the Mass Media."
6 Albert Cohen, cited in ibid., 316.
7 See for example Lewis and Ross, *Select Body*. The nature of the relation between drug use and HIV risk—whether causative, coincidental, or a socially acceptable explanation—has been consistently disputed. Weatherburn and SIGMA, "Alcohol Use and Unsafe Sexual Behaviour"; Rhodes, "Culture, Drugs and Unsafe Sex." Rises in the use of some substances, such as methamphetamine, for sexual purposes in gay cultures have been documented in North America and Australia. I discuss this issue further in chapter 7.
8 Keane, "Critiques of Harm Reduction, Morality and the Promise of Human Rights," 228.
9 Mugford, "Harm Reduction."
10 Ballard, "Constitution of AIDS," 132.
11 O'Malley and Valverde, "Pleasure, Freedom and Drugs," 36.
12 O'Malley, "Consuming Risks," 200.
13 Mauss, "Techniques of the Body," 461–62.
14 Mark Blasius, introductory note to Foucault, "About the Beginning of the Hermeneutics of the Self," 199.
15 Bennett, "Aestheticization of Ethics," 654.
16 As Bennett puts it, "These formulations exhibit a precise ambiguity with regard to the question of who or what is directing these 'elaborations' and 'operations' and what ends they serve." Ibid., 655.

17 Foucault, *Care of the Self*, 42. In fact, Foucault frames this research as an ethico-political response to the "type of individualization which is linked to the state." Foucault, "The Subject and Power."

18 For example, though Foucault questions the need for any "analytical or necessary link" between (sexual) ethics and social or political structures (Foucault, "On the Genealogy of Ethics," 261), in an interview in 1984 he says of sexuality, "It doesn't exist apart from a relationship to political structures, requirements, laws, and regulations that have a primary importance for it" (Foucault, "Polemics, Politics, and Problematizations," 114). In *The Use of Pleasure*, he speaks of the need to "keep in mind the distinction between the code elements of a morality and the elements of ascesis, neglecting neither their coexistence, their interrelations, their relative autonomy, nor their possible differences of emphasis" (31).

19 Foucault, *The Use of Pleasure*; Foucault, *Care of the Self*. For an extended theoretical elaboration of this point in relation to practices of harm reduction, see Race, "The Use of Pleasure in Harm Reduction."

20 Crimp, "How to Have Promiscuity in an Epidemic," 253.

21 Similarly, harm reduction practitioners recognized the presence of syringes within the habitus of intravenous drug use and made the provision of clean needles a priority.

22 From an article by William F. Buckley Jr. printed in the *New York Times* in 1986: "Everyone detected with AIDS should be tattooed in the upper forearm, to protect common-needle users, and on the buttocks, to prevent the victimization of other homosexuals." Quoted in Watney, *Policing Desire*, 44.

23 See Patton, *Inventing AIDS*; Kippax and Race, "Sustaining Safe Practice"; Ballard, "Constitution of AIDS."

24 Kippax and Race, "Sustaining Safe Practice."

25 Ibid., 6.

26 Kippax et al., "Sustaining Safe Sex."

27 P. Kinder, "A New Prevention Education Strategy for Gay Men: Responding to the Impact of AIDS on Gay Men's Lives" (paper presented at the XI International AIDS Conference, Vancouver, 1996). "Negotiated safety" allows for the discarding of condoms within seronegative regular relationships, so long as safe sex agreements are negotiated to cover sexual behavior outside these regular relationships, and HIV-testing has been conducted at appropriate intervals to ensure a reliable HIV-negative result. The educational slogan in Australia was "Talk, test, test, trust."

28 Van de Ven et al., "Increasing Proportions of Australian Gay and Homosexually Active Men Engage in Unprotected Anal Intercourse with Regular and Casual Partners."

29 Rosengarten, Race, and Kippax, *Touch Wood, Everything Will Be Okay*; Kip-

pax and Race, "Sustaining Safe Practice"; Race, "Revaluation of Risk among Gay Men."

30 Van de Ven et al., "In a Minority of Gay Men, Sexual Risk Practice Indicates Strategic Positioning for Perceived Risk Reduction Rather Than Unbridled Sex."

31 Van de Ven et al., "Increasing Proportions of Australian Gay and Homosexually Active Men Engage in Unprotected Anal Intercourse with Regular and Casual Partners."

32 See my overview in chapter 3. See also Morris, "Banality in Cultural Studies"; Frow, *Cultural Studies and Cultural Value*, chapter 2. This is one of the relative advantages of Foucault's ethics as a theoretical frame. While embodied ethics transfigure the social, they do not transcend it heroically in the way that some of the literature on pleasure and resistance seems to suggest.

33 Michel Foucault, "Sex, Power and the Politics of Identity," 165–66.

34 For a critical analysis of this in relation to Foucault's own work and homosexuality, see Halperin, *Saint Foucault*. See also Sedgwick, *Epistemology of the Closet*; Sedgwick, "Epidemics of the Will"; and Helen Keane's discussion of Betty Ford in Keane, *What's Wrong with Addiction?*, 82–84.

35 Frith, *Performing Rites*, 9. Similarly, John Frow argues that there is "no longer a stable hierarchy of value (even an inverted one) running from 'high' to 'low' culture, and that 'high' and 'low' culture can no longer, if they ever could, be neatly correlated with a hierarchy of social classes." Frow, *Cultural Studies and Cultural Value*, 1. He attributes this situation to the increased integration of aesthetic and economic production characteristic of the advanced capitalist world. For an application of notions of cultural capital to subcultural club culture, see Thornton, *Club Cultures*.

36 Frith, *Performing Rites*, 19.

37 Frith, *Performing Rites*, 4.

38 Ibid., 8.

39 Reynolds, "Through the Night," 71.

40 Walker, "Co-Dependent: Drugs and Australian Music," 156. One of the best depictions of the effect of a drug on a cultural scene is the portrayal in the film *24 Hour Party People* of the shift from punk to rave culture brought about, in part, by ecstasy (Michael Winterbottom, dir., 2002).

41 Walker, "Co-Dependent: Drugs and Australian Music," 162–63.

42 I develop this critique of the concept of "disinhibition" in chapter 7.

43 Reynolds, "Through the Night," 70.

44 Southgate and Hopwood, "Folk Pharmacology," 325.

45 Ibid.

46 Ibid.

47 It would be equally dangerous to believe that one can develop health strate-

gies from a position outside the play of value. Culture is not a homogenous mass, but a field of differentiation, and the freedom to differentiate between different sources of cultural value seems crucial. The enduring challenge is how to foster sentient practices of differentiation and safety without victimizing or demonizing certain parties.

48 Frith, *Performing Rites*, 13.

49 As Helen Keane conceives it, these interventions help to "constitute illicit drug users and addicts as people who are able to care for themselves (and others) and make decisions about their bodily practices." Keane, "Critiques of Harm Reduction," 231.

50 O'Malley and Valverde, "Pleasure, Freedom and Drugs," 36.

51 Ibid., 36, 37.

52 Ibid., 36–37.

53 Ibid., 36.

54 McInnes, Bollen, and Race, *Sexual Learning and Adventurous Sex*, 31.

55 I'm indebted here to Gay Hawkins's argument in "The Ethics of Television."

56 Patton, *Fatal Advice*, 139.

57 See, generally, Rose, *Inventing Our Selves*.

58 These particular resources are the product of qualitative inquiries conducted by educators and university-based cultural researchers trained in contemporary theories of sexuality and the body. I mention this point because this form of expertise is so frequently dismissed in the medical field. In the Australian context, the work of David McInnes and Jonathan Bollen has been particularly innovative and important in terms of advancing corporeal pedagogies in HIV education.

59 Note here that such initiatives always risk being linked to "taxpayer dollars" through the mechanism of state-funded "community-based organizations," even when they use independent funds to conduct more sensitive modes of education.

60 Watney, *Policing Desire*, 43.

61 Ballard, "Constitution of AIDS."

62 For an informative account of exactly these conditions as they affected the production of an ecstasy resource in the British context, see McDermott et al., "Ecstasy in the United Kingdom."

63 See McRobbie and Thornton, "Rethinking 'Moral Panic' for Multi-Mediated Social Worlds."

64 Fraser, quoted in Warner, *Publics and Counterpublics*, 118.

65 Ibid., 120, 121–22, 119.

66 Ibid., 116. Presumably, the gender specification is deliberate.

67 Ibid., 122.

68 Similarly, recent research in the HIV field argues that the "understanding of

sexual interaction as a learning environment must de-centre the primacy of message-based and information-providing approaches such as poster campaigns and printed resources such as booklets where such interventions assume a pre-emptive, self-defined self that once provided with information will act in appropriately healthy ways." McInnes, Bollen, and Race, *Sexual Learning and Adventurous Sex*, 31.

69 Warner develops this point in relation to gay men's HIV prevention in the final chapter of *Trouble with Normal*. See also Ballard, "Constitution of AIDS"; Dowsett, *Practising Desire*.

70 Indeed, many of the claims I make for these booklets can also be made for the booklet I discuss in chapter 4 (*Our Strongest Weapon Against Drugs . . . Families*), the difference being that the latter enjoys considerably more power to frame its address as the universal language of moral people.

71 Race, "Engaging in a Culture of Barebacking."

72 Too often, social analyses of health and medicine lose sight of the critical tension between the normative moral code and embodied ethics that can be found in Foucault's later work. The concept of "care of the self" has found much application in this literature, especially in relation to health and medicine, where it has been used analytically and empirically to characterize neoliberal regimes. To be sure, the terminology of "self" has had much purchase in a political climate where the self is cast as both the horizon and limit of social responsibility. But in taking "care of the self" to be emblematic of neoliberal regimes and rationalities in general, this literature evacuates this concept of much of its ethico-political momentum. Foucault developed this concept as part of a broader project that sought to counter the forms of totalization and individualization associated with the modern state. He wanted to show how in the Greco-Roman period the ethical question of "how to live" begins to turn on the notion of "care of the self" in a manner that was symptomatic of the growing tension between contemplative and practical knowledge. It is the individualizing effects of categorical knowledge that are the target of his critical efforts here. Foucault's ethics attempt to provide a basis for conceiving practical relations between care, pleasure, and knowledge that have some chance of resisting the prescriptive and demoralizing effects of official determinations of deviance. In short, "care of the self" cannot be equated with the exclusive, atomized self of neoliberal regimes—the *soi* of *le souci de soi* merely expresses a reflexive relation in being, not a thing called the self (though this point is often lost in translation). As Will McNeill puts it, Foucault's formulation of the ethical imperative to "care for the self" functions as a "historical imperative that formulates ethical existence as a task, as a relation to the future. 'Care for

yourself'—for whom? for what? who or what might that be? That is precisely the question." McNeill, "Care for the Self," 60. From this perspective, it would be a mistake to map "care for the self" uncritically onto the familiar neoliberal injunction (though this is a perfectly valid place to start). Against the diminished possibilities of this limited identification, Foucault offers a set of critical and historical tools that may be of assistance in trying to formulate one's existence as effectively as possible to respond ethically to the situation into which one is thrown. For further discussion of this point, see Race, "Queer Substances and Normative Substantiations."

7. Exceptional Sex

1 For discussions that frame drugs as an ethical rather than a moral problem, see Stengers and Ralet, "Drugs"; Keane, "Critiques of Harm Reduction"; Sybylla, "Hearing Whose Voice?"

2 This chapter is in part a response to Lauren Berlant's brilliant rethinking of agency in relation to sovereignty and embodiment. Berlant, "Slow Death (Sovereignty, Obesity, Lateral Agency)." I aim to put her highly original and important intervention and ideas into conversation with discussions of HIV, gay sex, and drug use.

3 See Fraser, " 'It's Your Life!' "; Race, "Engaging in a Culture of Barebacking"; O'Malley, "Consuming Risks."

4 Excellent critiques of given explanations of drug use in terms of social oppression, which nonetheless acknowledge systemic effects and structural pressures on agency, exist in Keane, "Women and Substance Abuse"; valentine and Fraser, "Trauma, Damage and Pleasure."

5 In the context of gay drug practices, see Green, "Chem Friendly." In an intelligent analysis, Green rejects social stigma and heterosexism as a sufficient explanation of gay drug practices, in favor of greater attention to the specificity of recreational drug use. However he ends up suggesting that drugs are used mainly as a form of self-medication to keep up with the exacting standards of the commercial gay scene and stranger sociability. This may be an accurate reflection of some people's perspectives, but the problem with this reading, in my view, is that it takes as given "natural" forms of intimacy (private, domestic, long-term)—and thus reproduces them—rather than querying these normative presumptions and highlighting alternative constructions (of sex, pleasure, and drug effects). See Berlant and Warner, "Sex in Public."

6 Keane, "Women and Substance Abuse," 77.

7 valentine and Fraser, "Trauma, Damage and Pleasure."

8 The most recent and appalling example of this in the Australian context is

the conservative former Prime Minister John Howard's use of the police and the military to intervene in the alleged problem of alcohol, drug, and child abuse within indigenous communities in the Northern Territory in 2007.

9 valentine and Fraser, "Trauma, Damage and Pleasure," 415. One of my favorite exercises with public health students is to have them read Philippe Bourgois's powerful ethnography of crack use in East Harlem, "Just Another Night in a Shooting Gallery." In this article, Bourgois tracks how the micro-practices of drug use within this population relate to entrenched structural violence of race, class, and poverty. In his concluding paragraph, he suggests that the "vitality of cultural expression [including music, dance, clothing, styles, and argot] on the poorest, most despised streets of the U.S. is best understood as an oppositional reaction to the conjugation of racism and unemployment." He suggests (not entirely unproblematically in my view) that the result of this alternative framework, when linked to drugs on the street, is "a self-destruction and community havoc that cements the status quo of gross socioeconomic inequality" (65). I ask students to think what a similar account might look like in relation to the forms of "recreational" drug use common in gay scenes ("Just Another Night on Manhunt"?). The exercise generates startling discussions around different notions of oppression, different attributions of agency and constraint, conceptions and practices of resistance, and conventional distinctions around drug practice and autonomous personhood, and their political and practical implications.

10 For a discussion of the intellectual risks of "insider" drug research, see Measham and Moore, "Reluctant Reflexivity."

11 Loss of full volitional control and self-sovereignty may of course make one vulnerable to exploitation by others—a point that has been used to legitimize forceful treatment of those deemed not to have sovereignty throughout history.

12 On the critical method of problematization, which obviously informs me extensively throughout, see Foucault, Use of Pleasure. See also my discussion and use of this method in chapters 2 and 3. For anthropological applications of "problematization," see Ong and Collier, Global Assemblages.

13 Halperin, What Do Gay Men Want? Halperin's work in general has enabled my thinking here in more ways than I can mention. For insight into the intensely moralized climate that surrounds HIV infection in the United States (much of it stirred up by gay conservative pundits), see the concluding chapter in Crimp, Melancholia and Moralism. Another brilliant and far-reaching intervention into questions of HIV, queer sex, moralism, and shame—which has informed much of my thinking around HIV and gay sex since its timely publication—is Warner, Trouble with Normal. Warner's coin-

ing of the phrase "the poppers effect"—the idea that with poppers you "give yourself a chance to swoon"—is the sort of insight that can inspire a whole project.

14 Halkitis, Parsons, and Stirratt, "A Double Epidemic."

15 For a good account of this, see Westacott, "Crystal-Meth."

16 See www.gaymeth.org (accessed 12 November 2007); www.caama.net (accessed 12 November 2007).

17 In community surveys conducted in gay urban centers like Sydney, around 20 percent of gay men in convenience samples report having used the drug in the last six months. In pooled data on methamphetamine use within the general population in Australia, daily use of the drug is confined to 2 percent of regular ecstasy users, and weekly use to 23 percent of this population, while these figures are halved again when it comes to frequency of use in the general youth population (twenty-two to twenty-nine years old). Degenhardt et al., "The Epidemiology of Methamphetamine Use and Harm in Australia." In a comparison of the drug practices of regular ecstasy users in Australia, both homosexual and heterosexual,there were higher general rates of crystal use among homosexual men in comparison to heterosexual men (64 percent versus 41 percent), but no differences in the median frequency of use (four days in the last six months). Homosexual men were however more likely to report "heavy" use of crystal than their heterosexual counterparts (defined as at least forty-five days in the last six months)—12 percent versus 2 percent—and had significantly higher median scores on a "Severity of Dependence" scale (two versus zero). Note however that under this definition of "heavy use," 52 percent of gay men in this sample report "non-heavy" use of crystal (over 80 percent of the gay crystal users). Homosexual men were however significantly more likely to report crystal was the primary form of methamphetamine about which they were concerned, and significantly more likely to report having injected drugs (26 percent versus 16 percent). Minimal differences existed between the groups in terms of reporting social, financial, work, or legal problems related to drug use generally: Fewer gay men reported work-related problems, while fewer heterosexual men reported social and financial problems. Degenhardt, "Drug Use and Risk Behaviour among Regular Ecstasy Users."

18 In this setting, the drug is often used in conjunction with GHB, which is said to have more sensual and dissociative effects.

19 For a beautiful example of such an undertaking, which reconfigures addiction as a form of intimacy, not just among people, but also with objects, see Keane, "Disorders of Desire." Keane draws on the groundbreaking critique of hegemonic intimacy found in Berlant and Warner, "Sex in Public."

20 In this context, gay community responses to new HIV infections have be-

come particularly condemnatory. See the discussion in the final chapter of Crimp, *Melancholia and Moralism.*

21 For more on how antidrug provisions have been used to patrol sexual minorities (among others) in history, see D. Osborne, *Suicide Tuesday*; Phongpaichit and Baker, *Thaksin*; Chauncey, *Gay New York*; Buckland, *Impossible Dance*; Slavin, "Crystal Methamphetamine Use among Gay Men in Sydney."

22 New South Wales Ombudsman, "Review of the Police Powers (Drug Detection Dogs) Act 2001," 2006; Bourgois, "Just Another Night in a Shooting Gallery."

23 Jarlais, "Intoxications, Intentions, and Disease Preventions."

24 Halkitis, Parsons, and Stirratt, "A Double Epidemic," 23.

25 J. Fortenberry et al., "Sex under the Influence"; Stall and Leigh, "Understanding the Relationship between Drug or Alcohol Use and High Risk Activity for HIV Transmission"; Weatherburn and SIGMA, "Alcohol Use and Unsafe Sexual Behaviour."; Leigh and Stall, "Substance Use and Risky Sexual Behavior for Exposure to HIV"; Rhodes and Stimson, "What Is the Relationship between Drug-Taking and Sexual Risk?"; Rhodes, "Culture, Drugs and Unsafe Sex"; Jarlais, "Intoxications, Intentions, and Disease Preventions"; Stall and Purcell, "Intertwining Epidemics"; Worth and Rawstorne, "Crystallizing the HIV Epidemic"; Gillmore et al., "Does 'High = High Risk'?"

26 Stall and Purcell, "Intertwining Epidemics"; Weatherburn, Davies, and Hickson, "No Connection between Alcohol Use and Unsafe Sex among Gay and Bisexual Men"; Gillmore et al., "Does 'High = High Risk'?"; Fortenberry et al., "Sex under the Influence"; Rhodes and Stimson, "What Is the Relationship between Drug-Taking and Sexual Risk?"

27 Halkitis, Shrem, and Martin, "Sexual Behavior Patterns of Methamphetamine-Using Gay and Bisexual Men."

28 Ibid. In multiple regression analyses, colleagues in Sydney have found that crystal use does not predict HIV infection among gay men outside the coincidence of a number of other variables which, combined, suggest participation in distinctive sex subcultures. Rawstorne and Worth, "Crystal Methamphetamine Use and Unsafe Sex"; Worth and Rawstorne, "Crystallizing the HIV Epidemic." This sociocultural interpretation is indicative of a crucial difference between Australian and U.S. mainstream HIV psychosocial research. Australian HIV social research has largely tried to avoid problematizing the "desires" of deviant groups, in favor of an approach that treats sex and drugs as social practice. See generally Race, "The Use of Pleasure in Harm Reduction." Obviously, the intervention of Heather Worth and Patrick Rawstorne has been pivotal for my analysis in this chapter.

29 MacAndrew and Edgerton, *Drunken Comportment*; Becker, *Outsiders*; Rhodes, "Culture, Drugs and Unsafe Sex."

30 Green, "Chem Friendly."

31 Green and Halkitis, "Crystal Methamphetamine and Sexual Sociality in an Urban Gay Subculture," 324.

32 Weatherburn and SIGMA, "Alcohol Use and Unsafe Sexual Behaviour"; Rhodes, "Culture, Drugs and Unsafe Sex."

33 Rhodes, "Culture, Drugs and Unsafe Sex," 756.

34 Westacott, "Crystal-Meth."

35 As mentioned, concerns around HIV transmission are obviously not the only motivating factor around anticrystal activism. There are many other problems associated, especially with heavy use. Part of the difficulty in some locations has been getting governments to provide adequate funding or support gay-specific programs around these various dangers *at all* without positing a direct connection to HIV transmission. Governments are unwilling to fund sexual-minority community-health initiatives that are not directly related to HIV prevention. Anticrystal activists and community-based organizations alike are thus put in the ignominious situation of having to endorse the notion of a direct causal link in order to get support for getting anything done on the issue at all. But as I am arguing, this move stands further to institutionalize an essentialized connection between crystal use and HIV risk in gay culture and discourse.

36 Halkitis, Parsons, and Stirratt, "A Double Epidemic," 25. Biology is sometimes cited here, specifically the negative effect of the drug on the ability to attain an erection. But gay users counter this effect with Viagra. At any rate, biochemical explanations deflect from a consideration of how norms of masculinity enter into gay men's lives to produce shame and pervasive disavowal of the pleasures of receptive anal sex. As an object of disinhibition discourse, crystal becomes available for facilitating, but also explaining away, passionate engagement in this practice.

37 In her study of gay crystal use in Los Angeles, Cathy Reback found that sexual subcommunities of crystal users have formed across class and ethnic differences. Cathy Reback, *The Social Construction of a Gay Drug: Methamphetamine Use among Gay and Bisexual Males in Los Angeles* (Los Angeles: City of Los Angeles AIDS Coordinator, 1997).

38 See, for example, the narratives of recovering users in Todd Ahlberg's film *Meth* (Babalu Pictures, 2005).

39 It is worth noting here that the forces that frown upon "illicit" sexual practice frequently turn for their support to a sort of HIV moralism that forgets —and is quite happy to promote a certain forgetting about—condoms. That is to say, the tendency is to conflate social deviance with HIV risk in a

manner that makes HIV prevention significantly less possible to enact or recognize in the context of "deviant" status. See Race, "Engaging in a Culture of Barebacking."

40 McKirnan, Ostrow, and Hope, "Sex, Drugs and Escape," 655.

41 Feminist cultural responses to binge eating have guided me here. These interventions provide an important model that rejects individualizing and psychological explanations of binge behavior in favor of an analysis of normative pressures, cultural material, and the experience of embodiment. See Bordo, *Unbearable Weight*.

42 Semple, Patterson, and Grant, "Motivations Associated with Methamphetamine Use among HIV+ Men Who Have Sex with Men"; Reback, "The Social Construction of a Gay Drug."

43 See Berlant, "Slow Death."

44 The experience of gay men here would seem to contrast significantly with the experience of rats, despite the resonances that some may find in the evocative title of a study by Anderson, Bignotto, and Tufik, "Facilitation of Ejaculation after Methamphetamine Administration in Paradoxical Sleep Deprived Rats." Prompted by the sexual reputation of methamphetamine, this study sets out to assess the effects of methamphetamine on sexual activity by giving paradoxical sleep deprived rats large doses of the drug and measuring their ejaculatory response over a sixty-minute period in a controlled trial, after which the rats were "killed by decapitation with a minimum of disturbance in an adjacent room." The researchers find that methamphetamine administration, in combination with sleep deprivation, does indeed make rats ejaculate at an increased rate over a sixty-minute period, thus "proving" the sexual reputation of methamphetamine. But in their own—apparently less "controlled"—experiments, gay men paradoxically find precisely the opposite (in relation to ejaculation).

45 Green and Halkitis, "Crystal Methamphetamine and Sexual Sociality in an Urban Gay Subculture."

46 Ibid., 323. See also Semple, Patterson, and Grant, "Motivations Associated with Methamphetamine Use."

47 Semple, Patterson, and Grant, "Motivations Associated with Methamphetamine Use."

48 Given the length of the HIV epidemic, and the ways it has worked its way into gay men's intimate lives to lace sex with anxiety and fear, this perspective may provide partial insight into both HIV-negative and HIV-positive gay men's use of substances in relation to sex. How much more magnified are these normative pressures for HIV-positive individuals in the context of recent initiatives in HIV education and legal enforcement which position

them as exclusively responsible for HIV transmission? The production of peer-based, sex-positive, nonmoralizing guidance on how to negotiate HIV-preventive sex from this social location should be a priority in my view. Such education would resonate with HIV-positive men's manifest concerns around HIV transmission. See Adam, "Constructing the Neoliberal Sexual Actor"; Race, "Engaging in a Culture of Barebacking."

49 Reback, "The Social Construction of a Gay Drug." For an excellent analysis of how this assumption plays out in HIV positive sexual cultures more generally, see Adam, "Constructing the Neoliberal Sexual Actor."

50 Semple, Patterson, and Grant, "Motivations Associated with Methamphetamine Use."

51 Reback, "The Social Construction of a Gay Drug."

52 Semple, Patterson, and Grant, "Motivations Associated with Methamphetamine Use," 153.

53 G. Leigh, "AIDS Inc. Uncovered," www.lifeormeth.org, ca. 2007, accessed 12 November 2007.

54 T. Valenzuela, "The Crystal Conundrum," *LA Weekly*, 9 June 2005.

55 Reback, "The Social Construction of a Gay Drug."

56 Purcell et al., "Illicit Substance Use, Sexual Risk, and HIV Positive Gay and Bisexual Men," S44.

57 For a more detailed analysis of practical ethics of HIV prevention that attempt to dispense with condoms, see Race, "Revaluation of Risk among Gay Men"; Race, "Engaging in a Culture of Barebacking"; Adam, "Constructing the Neoliberal Sexual Actor"; Rosengarten, Race, and Kippax, *Touch Wood, Everything Will Be Okay*.

58 I am indebted to one of my informants for coming up with the brilliant term *cracktivities* to describe the variation in drug-induced activities. Crystal methamphetamine is not the same substance as crack cocaine, but it is sometimes dubbed "crack" in gay vernacular, especially with reference to the glass pipe that is usually used for smoking it (the "crack pipe"). But of course this begs the question of what a "cracktive" analysis of crack cocaine would look like, and who can be supported to make such an intervention, and how. For an incisive critical analysis of how antidrug provisions have been used in the United States to deny and police black women's reproductive and corporeal autonomy in the name of the anticrack crusade, see Roberts, *Killing the Black Body*. For a good critical analysis of the televisual production of crack cocaine use in Reagan's America, see Reeves and Campbell, *Cracked Coverage*. For an anthropological analysis of drug use within severely marginalized communities that pays particular attention to the dynamics of sex and race, see Maher, *Sexed Work*. For further ethnographic

insight into structural constraints on agency in the context of racialized poverty and drug use, see the work of Philippe Bourgois, e.g., Bourgois, "Just Another Night in a Shooting Gallery."

59 The participant continues, "Sometimes tweaking can be good, and sometimes it's not good at all"—though the referents of this embodied evaluation of drug effects are ambiguous. Reback, "The Social Construction of a Gay Drug," 39.

60 Ibid., 38.

61 On contingent necessity and necessary contingency and the politics of recognizing being *as such*, see Agamben, *The Coming Community*.

62 Slavin, "Crystal Methamphetamine Use among Gay Men in Sydney."

63 These speculations are borne out in some of the data that Reback presents. One man talks about how he "always had a problem with integrating that part of me that likes to use crystal with the rest of my life. And, as a result, my life is very divided." Reback, "The Social Construction of a Gay Drug," 16. Another account shows how the adoption of addiction rhetoric makes one man unable to recognize the practical strategies *implicit in his own practice* that are serving to contain and moderate his use, in favor of a self-conception as hopeless and diseased. Reback, "The Social Construction of a Gay Drug," 22.

64 For a critique of employment-related drug testing and its maintenance of structural violence in relation to race and class, see O'Malley and Mugford, "Moral Technology."

65 For a more explicit, theoretically grounded elaboration of this method that attempts to engage the policy field, see Race, "The Use of Pleasure in Harm Reduction."

66 I am also aware that accounts of illicit agency and possibility are prone to be heroized or misread as statements of reified transgression or victorious sovereign intention. See Berlant, "Slow Death." I have been trying to work against this tendency while also trying to figure, as ontically as possible, specific formulations of hope or possibility. I guess another question arises here also: is it possible to have a response to a health problem that resists the forms of totalization and normative agency that would seem to be demanded by the policy sphere? Are *queer health* and *queer policy* oxymorons?

67 Hence the linguistic ontology of addiction. See note 63 above. And of course, see Derrida, "The Rhetoric of Drugs"; Ronnell, *Crack Wars*.

68 I would like to thank Lauren Berlant for taking me up on this point and pressing me for closure.

69 For a brilliant new analysis of theory on drugs, for example, see Boothroyd, *Culture on Drugs*. On the dense historicity of "losing oneself" and self-overcoming, see McNeill, "Care for the Self."

70 On "ethological" approaches and the ethicopolitical alternative they pro-
    vide to transcendent morality, see Deleuze, "Ethology." At the crux of an
    ethological approach to bodies is the insistence that we do not yet know
    what a body is capable of "in a given encounter, a given arrangement, a
    given combination." Deleuze, "Ethology," 627.
71 Sedgwick, "Epidemics of the Will."

SELECTED BIBLIOGRAPHY

...

Adam, Barry D. "Constructing the Neoliberal Sexual Actor: Responsibility and Care of the Self in the Discourse of Barebackers." *Culture, Health and Sexuality* 7, no. 4 (2005): 333–46.

Agamben, Giorgio. *The Coming Community.* Minneapolis: University of Minnesota Press, 1993.

——. *Homo Sacer: Sovereign Power and Bare Life.* Translated by Daniel Heller-Roazen. Stanford: Stanford University Press, 1995.

Allon, Fiona. "Nostalgia Unbound: Illegibility and the Synthetic Excess of Place." *Continuum* 14, no. 3 (2000): 275–87.

Amarasingham, Lorna. "Social and Cultural Perspectives on Medication Refusal." *American Journal of Psychiatry* 137, no. 3 (1980): 353–58.

Anderson, Monica, Magna Bignotto, and Sergio Tufik. "Facilitation of Ejaculation after Methamphetamine Administration in Paradoxical Sleep Deprived Rats." *Brain Research* 978, no. 1–2 (2003): 31–37.

Armstrong, David. "Clinical Autonomy, Individual and Collective: The Problem of Changing Doctors' Behaviour." *Social Science and Medicine* 55 (2002): 1771–77.

——. *The Political Anatomy of the Body: Medical Knowledge in Britain in the Twentieth Century.* Cambridge: Cambridge University Press, 1983.

Balint, Michael. *The Doctor, His Patient and the Illness.* Kent: Pitman Medical Publishing, 1957.

Ballard, John. "The Constitution of AIDS in Australia: Taking Government at a Distance Seriously." In *Governing Australia: Studies in Contemporary Rationalities of Government,* edited by Mitchell Dean and Barry Hindess, 125–38. Melbourne: Cambridge University Press, 1998.

Bardella, Claudio. "Pilgrimages of the Plagued: AIDS, Body and Society." *Body and Society* 8, no. 2 (2002): 79–105.

Bartos, Michael. "The Queer Excess of Public Health Policy." *Meanjin* 55, no. 1 (1996): 122–31.

Bartos, Michael, and Karalyn McDonald. "HIV as Identity, Experience or Career." *AIDS Care* 12, no. 3 (2000): 299–306.

Becker, Howard. *Outsiders: Studies in the Sociology of Deviance*. New York: Free Press, 1963.

Bell, Daniel. *The Cultural Contradictions of Capitalism*. London: Heinemann, 1976.

Benjamin, Walter. "The Work of Art in the Age of Mechanical Reproduction." In *Illuminations*, edited by Hannah Arendt, 219–53. England: Fontana, 1970.

Bennett, Jane. "'How Is It, Then, That We Still Remain Barbarians?' Foucault, Schiller, and the Aestheticization of Ethics." *Political Theory* 24, no. 4 (1996): 653–72.

Berlant, Lauren. *The Queen of America Goes to Washington City: Essays on Sex and Citizenship*. Durham, N.C.: Duke University Press, 1997.

———. "Slow Death (Sovereignty, Obesity, Lateral Agency)." *Critical Inquiry* 33 (2007): 754–80.

Berlant, Lauren, and Michael Warner. "Sex in Public." *Critical Inquiry* 24, no. 2 (1998): 547–66.

Berridge, Virginia, and Griffith Edwards. *Opium and the People: Opiate Use in Nineteenth Century England*. London: Allen Lane; New York: St Martin's, 1981.

Bersani, Leo. "Is the Rectum a Grave?" In *AIDS: Cultural Analysis, Cultural Activism*, edited by D. Crimp, 197–222. Cambridge, Mass.: MIT Press, 1988.

Bineham, Jeffery. "A Historical Account of the Hypodermic Model in Mass Communication." *Communication Monographs* 55 (1988): 230–49.

Bollen, Jonathan. "Sexing the Dance at Sleaze Ball 1994." *The Drama Review* 40, no. 3 (1996): 166–91.

Boothroyd, David. *Culture on Drugs: Narco-Cultural Studies of High Modernity*. Manchester: Manchester University Press, 2006.

Bordo, Susan. *Unbearable Weight: Feminism, Western Culture, and the Body*. Berkeley: University of California Press, 1993.

Bourgois, Philippe. "Just Another Night in a Shooting Gallery." *Theory, Culture and Society* 15, no. 2 (1998): 35–66.

Britain, Ian. "On Drugs." *Meanjin* 61, no. 2 (2002): 2–3.

Brown, Wendy. *States of Injury: Power and Freedom in Late Modernity*. Princeton: Princeton University Press, 1995.

Browne, Kevin, and Paul Freeling. *The Doctor-Patient Relationship*. Edinburgh: Churchill Livingstone, 1976.

Buckland, Fiona. *Impossible Dance: Club Culture and Queer World-Making*. Middletown, Conn.: Wesleyan University Press, 2002.

Butler, Judith. "Merely Cultural." *Social Text* 15, no. 52–53 (1997): 265–77.

Castiglia, Christopher. "Sex Panics, Sex Publics, Sex Memories." *Boundary* 27, no. 2 (2000): 149–72.

Chauncey, George. *Gay New York: Gender, Urban Culture and the Making of the Gay Male World, 1890–1940*. New York: Basic Books, 1994.

Clarke, John. *New Times and Old Enemies: Essays on Cultural Studies and America*. London: Harper Collins, 1991.

Connolly, William E. "Drugs, the Nation, and Freelancing: Decoding the Moral Universe of William Bennett." In *Drugs and the Limits of Liberalism: Moral and Legal Issues*, edited by Pablo DeGreiff, 173–212. Ithaca, N.Y.: Cornell University Press, 1999.

Conrad, Peter. "The Meaning of Medications: Another Look at Compliance." *Social Science and Medicine* 20, no. 1 (1985): 29–37.

Cot, Annie. "Neoconservative Economics, Utopia and Crisis." *Zone* 1–2 (1987): 293–311.

Coveney, John, and Robin Bunton. "In Pursuit of the Study of Pleasure: Implications for Health Research and Practice." *Health* 7, no. 2 (2003): 161–79.

Crawford, Robert. "The Boundaries of the Self and the Unhealthy Other: Reflections on Health, Culture and AIDS." *Social Science and Medicine* 38, no. 10 (1994): 1347–65.

Crimp, Douglas. "How to Have Promiscuity in an Epidemic." In *AIDS: Cultural Analysis/Cultural Activism*, edited by Crimp, 237–71. Cambridge, Mass.: MIT Press, 1988.

——. *Melancholia and Moralism: Essays on AIDS and Queer Politics*. Cambridge, Mass.: MIT Press, 2002.

Cvetkovich, Ann. *An Archive of Feelings: Trauma, Sexuality and Lesbian Public Cultures*. Durham, N.C.: Duke University Press, 2003.

Davidson, Arnold. "Foucault, Psychoanalysis and Pleasure." In *The Emergence of Sexuality*, 209–15. Cambridge, Mass.: Harvard University Press, 2001.

Davis, Milton. "Physiologic, Psychological and Demographic Factors in Patient Compliance with Doctors' Orders." *Medical Care* VI, no. 2 (1968): 115–22.

de Certeau, Michel. *The Practice of Everyday Life*. Berkley: University of California Press, 1984.

Degenhardt, Louise. "Drug Use and Risk Behaviour among Regular Ecstasy Users: Does Sexuality Make a Difference?" *Culture, Health and Sexuality* 7, no. 6 (2005): 599–614.

Degenhardt, L., A. Roxburgh, E. Black, R. Bruno, G. Campbell, S. Kinner, and J. Fetherston. "The Epidemiology of Methamphetamine Use and Harm in Australia." *Drug and Alcohol Review* 27 (2008): 243–52.

Delany, Samuel R. *The Motion of Light in Water: Sex and Science Fiction Writing in the East Village, 1957–1965*. New York: New American Library, 1988.

——. *Times Square Red, Times Square Blue*. New York: New York University Press, 1999.

Deleuze, Gilles. "Ethology: Spinoza and Us." In *Incorporations*, edited by Jonathan Crary and Sanford Kwinter, 625–33. New York: Zone Books, 1992.

Deleuze, Gilles, and Félix Guattari. *A Thousand Plateaus: Capitalism and Schizophrenia*. Translated by Brian Massumi. London: Althone, 1988.

Derrida, Jacques. "The Rhetoric of Drugs." In *Points: Interviews, 1974–1994*. Stanford: Stanford University Press, 1995.

Diprose, Rosalyn. *The Bodies of Women: Ethics, Embodiment, and Sexual Difference*. London: Routledge, 1994.

——. *Corporeal Generosity: On Giving with Nietzsche, Merleau-Ponty, and Levinas*. New York: State University of New York Press, 2002.

——. "The Hand That Writes Community in Blood." *Cultural Studies Review* 9, no. 1 (2003): 35–50.

Dixon, David. *From Prohibition to Regulation: Bookmaking, Anti-Gambling and the Law*. Oxford: Clarendon Press, 1991.

Donzelot, Jacques. *The Policing of Families*. Baltimore: Johns Hopkins University Press, 1997.

Dowsett, Gary. *Practising Desire: Homosexual Sex in the Era of AIDS*. Stanford: Stanford University Press, 1996.

Duggan, Lisa. *The Twilight of Equality? Neoliberalism, Cultural Politics, and the Attack on Democracy*. Boston: Beacon Press, 2003.

Dyer, Richard. "Judy Garland and Gay Men." In *Heavenly Bodies: Film Stars and Society*, 141–94. New York: St. Martin's, 1986.

Epstein, Steven. *Impure Science: AIDS, Activism and the Politics of Knowledge*. Berkeley: University of California Press, 1996.

Evans, David. *Sexual Citizenship: The Material Construction of Sexualities*. London: Routledge, 1993.

Featherstone, Mike. *Consumer Culture and Postmodernism*. London: Sage, 1991.

Flinn, Caryl. "The Deaths of Camp." In *Camp: Queer Aesthetics and the Performing Subject*, edited by Fabio Cleto, 433–57. Ann Arbor: University of Michigan Press, 1999.

Ford, Charles H., and Parker Tyler. *The Young and Evil*. Paris: Obelisk Press, 1933.

Fortenberry, J., D. Orr, B. Katz, E. Brizendine, and M. Blythe. "Sex under the Influence: A Diary Self-Report Study of Substance Use and Sexual Behavior among Adolescent Women." *Sexually Transmitted Diseases* 24, no. 6 (1997): 313–19.

Foucault, Michel. "About the Beginning of the Hermeneutics of the Self: Two Lectures at Dartmouth (Introductory Note from Mark Blasius)." *Political Theory* 21, no. 2 (1993): 198–227.

——. "The Birth of Biopolitics." In *Ethics: Subjectivity and Truth*, edited by Paul Rabinow, 73–80. London: Penguin, 1994.

———. *The Care of the Self: The History of Sexuality 3*. Translated by Robert Hurley. London: Penguin, 1990.

———. *The History of Sexuality, Volume 1: An Introduction*. Translated by Robert Hurley. London: Penguin, 1978.

———. "On the Genealogy of Ethics: An Overview of a Work in Progress." In *Ethics: Subjectivity and Truth*, edited by Paul Rabinow, 253–80. London: Penguin, 1997.

———. "Polemics, Politics, and Problematizations." In *Ethics: Subjectivity and Truth*, edited by Paul Rabinow, 111–20. London: Penguin, 1997.

———. "Sex, Power and the Politics of Identity." In *Ethics: Subjectivity and Truth*, edited by Paul Rabinow, 163–74. London: Penguin, 1997.

———. "The Subject and Power." In *Michel Foucault: Beyond Structuralism and Hermeneutics*, edited by Hubert L. Dreyfus and Paul Rabinow, 208–26. New York: Harvester Wheatsheaf, 1982.

———. *The Use of Pleasure: The History of Sexuality 2*. Translated by Robert Hurley. Vol. 2. London: Penguin, 1984.

Fraser, Suzanne. "'It's Your Life!': Injecting Drug Users, Individual Responsibility and Hepatitis C Prevention." *Health*, no. 8 (2004): 199–221.

Friedman, Milton, and Rose Friedman. *The Tyranny of the Status Quo*. San Diego: Harcourt Brace Jovanovich, 1984.

Frith, Simon. *Performing Rites: On the Value of Popular Music*. London: Oxford University Press, 1996.

Frow, John. *Cultural Studies and Cultural Value*. London: Oxford University Press, 1995.

———. "Cultural Studies and the Neoliberal Imagination." *Yale Journal of Criticism* 12, no. 2 (2000): 424–30.

Gatens, Moira. *Imaginary Bodies: Ethics, Power and Corporeality*. London: Routledge, 1996.

Gibbs, Anna. "Contagious Feelings: Pauline Hanson and the Epidemiology of Affect." *Australian Humanities Review* 21 (December 2001). http://www.australianhumanitiesreview.org.

Gillmore, Mary, Diane Morrison, Barbara Leigh, Marilyn Hoppe, Jan Gaylord, and Damian Rainey. "Does 'High = High Risk'? An Event-Based Analysis of the Relationship between Substance Use and Unprotected Anal Sex among Gay and Bisexual Men." *AIDS and Behavior* 6, no. 4 (2002): 361–70.

Gilroy, Paul. *The Black Atlantic*. London: Verso, 1993.

Goddard, Martyn. "AIDS in Never-Never Land." *National AIDS Bulletin* 14, no. 4 (2001): 26–27.

Green, Adam. "Chem Friendly: The Institutional Basis of Club Drug Use in a Sample of Urban Gay Men." In *Drugs, Clubs and Young People: Sociological* and Public Health Perspectives, edited by Bill Sanders, 67–76. Burlington, Vt.: Ashgate, 2006.

Green, Adam, and Perry Halkitis. "Crystal Methamphetamine and Sexual Sociality in an Urban Gay Subculture: An Elective Affinity." Culture, Health and Sexuality 8, no. 4 (2006): 317–33.

Grosz, Elizabeth. Volatile Bodies: Toward a Corporeal Feminism. Bloomington: Indiana University Press, 1994.

Hage, Ghassan. "The Incredible Shrinking Society." Financial Review, 7 September 2001.

——. White Nation: Fantasies of White Supremacy in a Multicultural Society. Sydney: Pluto Press, 2000.

Halberstam, Judith. In a Queer Time and Place: Transgender Bodies, Subcultural Lives. New York: New York University Press, 2005.

Halkitis, Perry, Jeff Parsons, and Michael Stirratt. "A Double Epidemic: Crystal Methamphetamine Drug Use in Relation to HIV Transmission among Gay Men." Journal of Homosexuality 41, no. 2 (2001): 17–35.

Halkitis, Perry, Michael T. Shrem, and Frederick Martin. "Sexual Behavior Patterns of Methamphetamine-Using Gay and Bisexual Men." Substance Use and Misuse 40 (2005): 703–19.

Hall, Stuart. The Hard Road to Renewal: Thatcherism and the Crisis of the Left. London: Verso, 1988.

——. "Notes on Deconstructing 'the Popular.'" In People's History and Socialist Theory, edited by Raphael Samuel, 227–39. London: Routledge and Kegan Paul, 1981.

——. "Reformism and the Legislation of Consent." In Permissiveness and Control: The Fate of the Sixties Legislation, edited by National Deviancy Conference, 1–43. London: Macmillan, 1980.

Hall, Stuart, and Tony Jefferson, eds. Resistance through Rituals: Youth Subcultures in Post-War Britain. London: Hutchinson, 1976.

Halperin, David. "Homosexuality's Closet." Michigan Quarterly Review 41, no. 1 (2002): 21–53.

——. How to Do the History of Homosexuality. Chicago: University of Chicago Press, 2002.

——. Saint Foucault. Oxford: Oxford University Press, 1995.

——. What Do Gay Men Want? An Essay on Sex, Risk and Subjectivity. Ann Arbor: University of Michigan Press, 2007.

Haraway, Donna. "A Cyborg Manifesto: Science, Technology, and Socialist-Feminism in the Late Twentieth Century." In Simians, Cyborgs, and Women: The Reinvention of Nature, 149–81. New York: Routledge, 1991.

——. "Situated Knowledges: The Science Question in Feminism and the Privilege of Partial Perspective." In *Simians, Cyborgs, and Women: The Reinvention of Nature*, 183–201. New York: Routledge, 1991.

Hardt, Michael, and Antonio Negri. *Empire*. Cambridge, Mass.: Harvard University Press, 2000.

Hawkins, Gay. "The Ethics of Television." *International Journal of Cultural Studies* 4, no. 4 (2001): 412–26.

Haynes, R. Brian, David L. Sackett, and D. Wayne Taylor, eds. *Compliance in Health Care*. Baltimore: Johns Hopkins University Press, 1979.

Hebdige, Dick. *Subculture: The Meaning of Style*. London: Methuen, 1979.

Henderson, Saras, and Alan Petersen. *Consuming Health: The Commodification of Health Care*. London: Routledge, 2002.

Himmelstein, Jerome L. "From Killer Weed to Drop-out Drug: The Changing Ideology of Marijuana." *Contemporary Crises* 7 (1983): 13–38.

Holleran, Andrew. *Dancer from the Dance: A Novel*. New York: William Morrow, 1978.

Hurley, Michael. "Sydney." In *Queer City: Gay and Lesbian Politics in Sydney*, edited by Craig Johnston and Paul van Reyk, 241–57. Sydney: Pluto Press, 2001.

James, John S. "Protease Inhibitors' Metabolic Side-Effects: Cholesterol, Triglycerides, Blood Sugar, and 'Crix Belly.'" *AIDS Treatment News* 277 (1997). http://www.aids.org/atn/a-277–01.html.

Jarlais, Don. "Intoxications, Intentions, and Disease Preventions." *Sexually Transmitted Diseases* 24, no. 6 (1997): 320–21.

Keane, Helen. "Critiques of Harm Reduction, Morality and the Promise of Human Rights." *International Journal of Drug Policy* 14, no. 3 (2003): 227–32.

——. "Disorders of Desire: Addiction and Problems of Intimacy." *Journal of Medical Humanities* 25, no. 3 (2004): 189–204.

——. *What's Wrong with Addiction?* Melbourne: Melbourne University Press, 2002.

——. "Women and Substance Abuse: Problems of Visibility and Empowerment." In *Women's Health: Contemporary International Perspectives*, edited by Jane M. Ussher, 76–82. Leicester: British Psychological Society, 2000.

Keane, Helen, and Marsha Rosengarten. "On the Biology of Sexed Subjects." *Australian Feminist Studies* 17, no. 39 (2002): 261–77.

Kipnis, Laura. "(Male) Desire and (Female) Disgust: Reading *Hustler*." In *Cultural Studies*, edited by Lawrence Grossberg, Cary Nelson, and Paula A. Treichler, 373–91. New York: Routledge, 1992.

Kippax, Susan. "Sexual Health Interventions Are Unsuitable for Experimental Evaluation." In *Effective Sexual Health Interventions: Issues in Experimental Evaluation*, edited by Judith M. Stephenson, John Imrie, and Chris Bonell, 17–34. Oxford: Oxford University Press, 2003.

Kippax, Susan, June Crawford, Mark Davis, Pam Rodden, and Gary Dowsett. "Sustaining Safe Sex: A Longitudinal Study of a Sample of Homosexual Men." *AIDS* 7 (1993): 257–63.

Kippax, Susan, and Kane Race. "Sustaining Safe Practice: Twenty Years On." *Social Science and Medicine* 57 (2003): 1–12.

Kippax, Susan, and Paul Van de Ven. "An Epidemic of Orthodoxy? Design and Methodology in the Evaluation of the Effectiveness of HIV Health Promotion." *Critical Public Health* 8 (1998): 371–86.

Kramer, Peter. *Listening to Prozac.* London: Fourth Estate, 1994.

Latour, Bruno. *We Have Never Been Modern.* Cambridge, Mass.: Harvard University Press, 1993.

Law, Matthew G., Li Yeuming, A. M. McDonald, D. Cooper, and J. Kaldor. "Estimating the Population Impact in Australia of Improved Antiviral Treatment for HIV Infection." *AIDS* 14 (2000): 197–201.

Leigh, Barbara, and Ron Stall. "Substance Use and Risky Sexual Behavior for Exposure to HIV: Issues in Methodology, Interpretation, and Prevention." *American Psychology* 48 (1993): 1035–45.

Lerner, Barron. "From Careless Consumptives to Recalcitrant Patients: The Historical Construction of Noncompliance." *Social Science and Medicine* 45, no. 9 (1997): 1423–31.

Levine, Harry G. "The Discovery of Addiction: Changing Conceptions of Habitual Drunkenness in America." *Journal of Studies on Alcohol* 39, no. 1 (1978): 143–74.

———. "Global Drug Prohibition: Its Uses and Crises." *International Journal of Drug Policy* 14, no. 2 (2003): 145–53.

Lewis, Lynette, and Michael Ross. *A Select Body: The Gay Dance Party Subculture and the HIV/AIDS Pandemic.* New York: Cassell, 1995.

MacAndrew, Craig, and Robert Edgerton. *Drunken Comportment: A Social Explanation.* Chicago: Aldine, 1969.

Maher, Lisa. *Sexed Work: Gender, Race and Resistance in a Brooklyn Drug Market.* Oxford: Clarendon Press, 1997.

Manderson, Desmond. "The Semiotics of the Title: A Comparative and Historical Analysis of Drug Legislation." *Law/Text/Culture* 2 (1995): 160–77.

Marks, Harry. "Revisiting the Origins of Compulsory Drug Prescriptions." *American Journal of Public Health* 85, no. 1 (1995): 109–15.

Martin, Biddy. *Femininity Played Straight: The Significance of Being Lesbian.* New York: Routledge, 1997.

Mauss, Marcel. "Techniques of the Body." 1934. In *Incorporations*, edited by Jonathan Crary and Sanford Kwinter, 454–77. New York: Zone, 1992.

McCormack, G. "Marijuana Smoking Seen as Epidemic among the Idle." *Science News Letter* 34 (1938): 340.

McDermott, P., A. Matthews, P. O'Hare, and A. Bennett. "Ecstasy in the United Kingdom: Recreational Drug-Use and Subcultural Change." In *Psychoactive Drugs and Harm Reduction: From Faith to Science*, edited by Nick Heather, Alex Wodak, Ethan Nadelmann, and Pat O'Hare, 230–46. London: Whurr, 1993.

McGregor, Fiona. *Chemical Palace*. Crows Nest, NSW: Allen and Unwin, 2002.

McInnes, David, Jonathan Bollen, and Kane Race. *Sexual Learning and Adventurous Sex*. Sydney: School of Humanities, University of Western Sydney, 2002.

McKirnan, David, D. Ostrow, and B. Hope. "Sex, Drugs and Escape: A Psychological Model of HIV-Risk Sexual Behaviours." *AIDS Care* 8, no. 6 (1996): 655–69.

McNeill, Will. "Care for the Self: Originary Ethics in Heidegger and Foucault." *Philosophy Today* 42 (1998): 53–64.

McQuire, Scott. "From Glass Architecture to Big Brother: Scenes from a Cultural History of Transparency." *Cultural Studies Review* 9, no. 1 (2003): 103–23.

McRobbie, Angela, and Sarah Thornton. "Rethinking 'Moral Panic' for Multi-Mediated Social Worlds." *British Journal of Sociology* 46, no. 4 (1995): 559–74.

Measham, Fiona, and Karenza Moore. "Reluctant Reflexivity: Implicit Insider Knowledge and the Development of Club Studies." In *Drugs, Clubs and Young People: Sociological and Public Health Perspectives*, edited by Bill Sanders, 13–25. Burlington, Vt.: Ashgate, 2006.

Metzl, Jonathan. "If Direct-to-Consumer Advertisements Come to Europe: Lessons from the USA." *Lancet* 369, no. 9562 (2007): 704–6.

Michaels, Eric. "Carnivale in Oxford St." *New Theatre*, May–June (1988): 4–8.

Morgan, H. Wayne. *Drugs in America: A Social History, 1800–1980*. New York: Syracuse University Press, 1981.

Morris, Meaghan. "Banality in Cultural Studies." In *Logics of Television: Essays in Cultural Criticism*, edited by Patricia Mellencamp, 14–43. Bloomington: Indiana University Press, 1990.

———. "'Please Explain?' Ignorance, Poverty and the Past." *Inter-Asia Cultural Studies* 1, no. 2 (2000): 219–32.

———. *Too Soon Too Late: History in Popular Culture*. Bloomington: Indiana University Press, 1998.

Morrison, Paul. *The Explanation for Everything: Essays on Sexual Subjectivity*. New York University: New York University Press, 2001.

Morse, Margaret. "An Ontology of Everyday Distraction." In *Logics of Television: Essays in Cultural Criticism*, edited by Patricia Mellencamp, 193–221. Bloomington: Indiana University Press, 1990.

Moynihan, Ray. "The Making of a Disease: Female Sexual Dysfunction." *BMJ* 326 (2003): 45–47.

Moynihan, Ray, and David Henry, eds. "Disease Mongering." Special issue, *PLOS Medicine* 3, no. 4 (2006).

Mugford, Stephen. "Harm Reduction: Does It Lead to Where Its Proponents Imagine?" In *Psychoactive Drugs and Harm Reduction: From Faith to Science*, edited by Nick Heather, Alex Wodak, Ethan Nadelmann, and Pat O'Hare, 21–33. London: Whurr, 1993.

Mulvey, Laura. "Some Thoughts on Theories of Fetishism in the Context of Contemporary Culture." *October* 65 (1993): 3–20.

Musto, David. *The American Disease: Origins of Narcotics Control.* New Haven: Yale University Press, 1973.

Nabarro, David. "The Defaulting Child." *British Journal of Venereal Diseases* 11 (1935): 91–97.

Nicoll, Fiona. *From Diggers to Drag Queens: Configurations of Australian National Identity.* Sydney: Pluto Press, 2001.

Olmo, Rosa del. "The Hidden Face of Drugs." *Social Justice: A Journal of Crime, Conflict and World Order* 18 (1991): 10–48.

O'Malley, Pat. "Consuming Risks: Harm Minimization and the Government of 'Drug-Users.'" In *Governable Places: Readings on Governmentality and Crime Control*, edited by Russell Smandych, 191–214. Aldershot, U.K.: Dartmouth, 1999.

———. "Containing Our Excitement: Commodity Culture and the Crisis of Discipline." *Studies in Law, Politics and Society* 13 (1993): 159–86.

———. "Risk and Responsibility." In *Foucault and Political Reason: Liberalism, Neo-Liberalism and Rationalities of Government*, edited by Andrew Barry, Thomas Osborne, and Nikolas Rose, 189–208. London: UCL Press, 1996.

O'Malley, Pat, and Stephen Mugford. "The Demand for Intoxicating Commodities: Implications for the 'War on Drugs.'" *Social Justice: A Journal of Crime, Conflict and World Order* 18 (1992): 49–75.

———. "Moral Technology: The Political Agenda of Random Drug Testing." *Social Justice: A Journal of Crime, Conflict and World Order* 18 (1991): 122–46.

O'Malley, Pat, and Mariana Valverde. "Pleasure, Freedom and Drugs: The Uses of 'Pleasure' in Liberal Governance of Drug and Alcohol Consumption." *Sociology* 38, no. 1 (2004): 25–42.

Ong, Aihwa, and Stephen J. Collier. *Global Assemblages: Technology, Politics, and Ethics as Anthropological Problems.* Oxford: Wiley-Blackwell, 2004.

Osborne, Duncan. *Suicide Tuesday: Gay Men and the Crystal Meth Scare.* New York: Carroll and Graf, 2005.

Osborne, Thomas. "Power and Persons: On Ethical Stylisation and Person-Centred Medicine." *Sociology of Health and Illness* 16, no. 4 (1994): 515–35.

Patton, Cindy. *Fatal Advice: How Safe Sex Education Went Wrong*. Durham, N.C.: Duke University Press, 1996.

———. *Inventing AIDS*. New York: Routledge, 1990.

Persson, Asha, Kane Race, and Elizabeth Wakeford. "HIV Health in Context: Negotiating Medical Technology and Lived Experience." *Health* 7, no. 4 (2003): 397–415.

Phongpaichit, Pasuk, and Christopher Baker. *Thaksin: The Business of Politics in Thailand*. Bangkok: Silkworm Books, 2004.

Povinelli, Elizabeth. *The Empire of Love: Toward a Theory of Intimacy, Genealogy and Carnality*. Durham, N.C.: Duke University Press, 2006.

Pozniak, Anton. "Surrogacy in HIV-1 Clinical Trials." *Lancet* 351, no. 9102 (1998): 536–37.

Probyn, Elspeth. *Blush: Faces of Shame*. Sydney: University of New South Wales Press, 2005.

———. *Sexing the Self: Gendered Positions in Cultural Studies*. London: Routledge, 1993.

Purcell, Daniel, S. Moss, R. Remien, W. Woods, and J. Parsons. "Illicit Substance Use, Sexual Risk, and HIV Positive Gay and Bisexual Men: Differences by Serostatus of Casual Partners." *AIDS* 19, no. S1 (2005): S37–47.

Race, Kane. "Engaging in a Culture of Barebacking: Gay Men and the Risk of HIV Prevention." In *Gendered Risks*, edited by Kelly Hannah-Moffat and Pat O'Malley, 99–126. London: Routledge, 2007.

———. "Incorporating Clinical Authority: A New Test for People with HIV." In *Reframing the Body*, edited by Nick Watson and Sarah Cunningham-Burley, 81–95. Hampshire: Palgrave, 2001.

———. "Queer Substances and Normative Substantiations: Of Drugs, Dogs, and Other Piggy Practices." In *Queer Somatechnics*, edited by N. Sullivan and S. Murray. London: Ashgate, forthcoming.

———. "Revaluation of Risk among Gay Men." *AIDS Education and Prevention* 15, no. 4 (2003): 369–81.

———. "The Undetectable Crisis: Changing Technologies of Risk." *Sexualities* 4, no. 2 (2001): 167–89.

———. "The Use of Pleasure in Harm Reduction: Perspectives from the History of Sexuality." *International Journal of Drug Policy* 19, no. 5 (2008): 417–23.

Race, Kane, and Elizabeth Wakeford. "Dosing on Time: Developing Adherent Practice with Highly Active Antiretroviral Therapy." *Culture, Health and Sexuality* 2, no. 2 (2000): 213–28.

Rasmussen, Nicolas. "Making the First Anti-Depressant: Amphetamine in American Medicine 1929–1950." *Journal of the History of Medicine and Allied Sciences* 61, no. 3 (2006): 288–323.

Rawstorne, Patrick, and Heather Worth. "Crystal Methamphetamine Use and Unsafe Sex." *HIV Australia* 3, no. 4 (2004): 14–16.

Redhead, Steve. *Rave Off: Politics and Deviance in Contemporary Youth Culture.* Avebury: Aldershot, 1993.

Reeves, Jimmie, and Richard Campbell. *Cracked Coverage: Television News, the Anti-Cocaine Crusade, and the Reagan Legacy.* Durham, N.C.: Duke University Press, 1994.

Reynolds, Robert. "Through the Night." *Meanjin* 61, no. 2 (2002): 67–73.

Rhodes, Tim. "Culture, Drugs and Unsafe Sex: Confusion About Causation." *Addiction* 91, no. 6 (1996): 753–58.

Rhodes, Tim, and Gerry Stimson. "What Is the Relationship between Drug-Taking and Sexual Risk? Social Relations and Social Research." *Sociology of Health and Illness* 16 (1994): 209–29.

Roberts, Dorothy. *Killing the Black Body: Race, Reproduction and the Meaning of Liberty.* New York: Pantheon, 1997.

Rofes, Eric. *Dry Bones Breathe: Gay Men Creating Post-AIDS Identities and Cultures.* Binghampton: Harrington Park, 1998.

Ronnell, Avital. *Crack Wars: Literature, Addiction, Mania.* Nebraska: University of Nebraska Press, 1992.

Rose, Nikolas. "Government, Authority and Expertise in Advanced Liberalism." *Economy and Society* 22, no. 3 (1993): 283–99.

——. *Inventing Our Selves: Psychology, Power and Personhood.* Cambridge: Cambridge University Press, 1998.

——. "The Politics of Life Itself." *Theory, Culture and Society* 18, no. 6 (2001): 1–30.

Rosengarten, Marsha. "Consumer Activism in the Pharmacology of HIV." *Body and Society* 10, no. 1 (2004): 91–107.

——. *HIV Interventions: Biomedicine and the Traffic between Information and Flesh.* Seattle: University of Washington Press, forthcoming.

Rosengarten, Marsha, Kane Race, and Susan Kippax. *Touch Wood, Everything Will Be Okay: Gay Men's Understandings of Clinical Markers in Sexual Practice.* Sydney: National Centre in HIV Social Research, University of New South Wales, 2000.

Rosenstock, Irwin. "Patients' Compliance with Health Regimens." *JAMA* 234, no. 4 (1975): 402–3.

Ross, Andrew. "Epilogue: Calculating the Risk." In *Policing Public Sex*, edited by Dangerous Bedfellows, 395–400. Boston: South End, 1996.

——. *No Respect: Intellectuals and Popular Culture.* New York: Routledge, 1989.

Roth, H., H. Caron, and P. Bartholomew. "Measuring Intake of a Prescribed Medication: A Bottle Count and a Tracer Technique Compared." *Clinical Pharmacology and Therapeutics* 11, no. 2 (1970): 228–37.

Royal Pharmaceutical Society of Great Britain. *From Compliance to Concordance: Achieving Shared Goals in Medicine Taking*. London: Royal Pharmaceutical Society of Great Britain, 1997.

Rundle, Guy. "The Opportunist: John Howard and the Triumph of Reaction." *Quarterly Essay* 3 (2001).

Sackett, David L., and R. Brian Haynes. *Compliance with Therapeutic Regimens*. Baltimore: Johns Hopkins University Press, 1976.

Sanders, Bill, ed. *Drugs, Clubs and Young People: Sociological and Public Health Perspectives*. Burlington, Vt.: Ashgate, 2006.

Saunders, Nicholas. *Ecstasy and the Dance Culture*. Exeter: BPC Wheatons, 1995.

Scott, Joan. "Experience." In *Feminists Theorize the Political*, edited by Judith Butler and Joan Scott, 22–40. New York: Routledge, 1992.

Sedgwick, Eve Kosofsky. "Epidemics of the Will." In *Tendencies*, 130–42. Durham, N.C.: Duke University Press, 1993.

———. *Epistemology of the Closet*. London: Penguin, 1990.

———. "Paranoid Reading and Reparative Reading: Or, You're So Paranoid, You Probably Think This Introduction Is About You." In *Novel Gazing: Queer Readings in Fiction*, edited by Sedgwick, 1–40. Durham, N.C.: Duke University Press, 1997.

———. *Touching Feeling: Affect, Pedagogy, Performativity*. Durham, N.C.: Duke University Press, 2003.

Semple, Shirley, T. L. Patterson, and I. Grant. "Motivations Associated with Methamphetamine Use among HIV+ Men Who Have Sex with Men." *Journal of Substance Abuse Treatment* 22 (2002): 149–56.

Sendziuk, Paul. *Learning to Trust: Australian Responses to AIDS*. Sydney: University of New South Wales Press, 2003.

Simon, Jonathan. "The Emergence of a Risk Society: Insurance, Law and the State." *Socialist Review* 95 (1987): 61–89.

Slavin, Sean. "Crystal Methamphetamine Use among Gay Men in Sydney." *Contemporary Drug Problems* 31, no. 3 (2004): 425–65.

Sontag, Susan. "Notes on 'Camp.'" In *Camp: Queer Aesthetics and the Performing Subject*, edited by Fabio Cleto, 53–65. Ann Arbor: University of Michigan Press, 1999.

Southgate, Erica, and Max Hopwood. "Mardi Gras Says 'Be Drug Free': Accounting for Resistance, Pleasure and the Demand for Illicit Drugs." *Health* 3, no. 3 (1999): 303–16.

———. "The Role of Folk Pharmacology and Lay Experts in Harm Reduction: Sydney Gay Drug Using Networks." *International Journal of Drug Policy* 12, no. 4 (2001): 321–35.

Spigel, Lynn. "Television in the Family Circle: The Popular Reception of a New

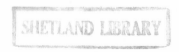
SHETLAND LIBRARY

Medium." In *Logics of Television: Essays in Cultural Criticism*, edited by Patricia Mellencamp, 73–97. Bloomington: Indiana University Press, 1990.

Stall, Ron, and Barbara Leigh. "Understanding the Relationship between Drug or Alcohol Use and High Risk Activity for HIV Transmission: Where Do We Go from Here?" *Addiction* 89 (1994): 149–52.

Stall, Ron, and David W. Purcell. "Intertwining Epidemics: A Review of Research on Substance Use among Men Who Have Sex with Men and Its Connection to the AIDS Epidemic." *AIDS and Behavior* 4, no. 2 (2000): 181–92.

Stengers, Isabelle, and Olivier Ralet. "Drugs: Ethical Choice or Moral Consensus?" In *Power and Invention: Situating Science*, 215–32. Minneapolis: Minnesota University Press, 1997.

Stimson, Gerry. "Obeying Doctor's Orders: A View from the Other Side." *Social Science and Medicine* 8 (1972): 97–104.

Stone, Sandy. "The Empire Strikes Back: A Posttransexual Manifesto." 1991. In *The Transgender Studies Reader*, edited by Susan Stryker and Stephen Whittle, 221–35. New York: Routledge, 2006.

Stryker, Susan, and Stephen Whittle, eds. *The Transgender Studies Reader*. New York: Routledge, 2006.

Sybylla, Roe. "Hearing Whose Voice? The Ethics of Care and the Practices of Liberty." *Economy and Society* 30, no. 1 (2001): 66–84.

Temin, Peter. *Taking Your Medicine: Drug Regulation in the United States*. Cambridge, Mass.: Harvard University Press, 1980.

Thornton, Sarah. *Club Cultures: Music, Media and Subcultural Capital*. London: Polity, 1995.

Torres, Sasha. "The Caped Crusader of Camp: Pop, Camp, and the Batman Television Series." In *Camp: Queer Aesthetics and the Performing Subject*, edited by Fabio Cleto, 330–43. Ann Arbor: University of Michigan Press, 1999.

Treloar, Carla, and Martin Holt, eds. "Pleasure and Drugs." Special issue, *International Journal of Drug Policy* 19, no. 5 (2008).

Trostle, James. "Medical Compliance as an Ideology." *Social Science and Medicine* 27, no. 12 (1988): 1299–308.

Trouiller, Patrice, P. Olliaro, E. Torreele, and J. Orbinski. "Drug Development for Neglected Diseases: A Deficient Market and a Public Health Policy Failure." *Lancet* 359, no. 9324 (2002): 2188–94.

valentine, kylie, and Suzanne Fraser. "Trauma, Damage and Pleasure: Rethinking Problematic Drug Use." *International Journal of Drug Policy* 19, no. 5 (2008): 410–16.

Valverde, Mariana. "'Despotism' and Ethical Liberal Governance." *Economy and Society* 25, no. 3 (1996): 357–72.

Van de Ven, Paul, Susan Kippax, June Crawford, Patrick Rawstorne, Garrett

Prestage, Andrew Grulich, and Dean Murphy. "In a Minority of Gay Men, Sexual Risk Practice Indicates Strategic Positioning for Perceived Risk Reduction Rather Than Unbridled Sex." *AIDS Care* 14 (2002): 471–80.

Van de Ven, Paul, Patrick Rawstorne, June Crawford, and Susan Kippax. "Increasing Proportions of Australian Gay and Homosexually Active Men Engage in Unprotected Anal Intercourse with Regular and Casual Partners." *AIDS Care* 14 (2002): 335–41.

Walker, Clinton. "Co-Dependent: Drugs and Australian Music." *Meanjin* 61, no. 2 (2002): 154–75.

Warner, Michael. "Liberalism and the Cultural Studies Imagination: A Comment on John Frow." *Yale Journal of Criticism* 12, no. 2 (1999): 431–33.

——. *Publics and Counterpublics*. New York: Zone Books, 2002.

——. *The Trouble with Normal: Sex, Politics and the Ethics of Queer Life*. Cambridge, Mass.: Harvard University Press, 1999.

Watkins, Elizabeth. *On the Pill: A Social History of Oral Contraceptives, 1950–1970*. Baltimore: Johns Hopkins University Press, 1998.

Watney, Simon. *Policing Desire: Pornography, AIDS and the Media*. London: Methuen, 1987.

Weatherburn, Peter, Peter Davies, and Ford Hickson. "No Connection between Alcohol Use and Unsafe Sex among Gay and Bisexual Men." *AIDS* 7 (1993): 115–19.

Weatherburn, Peter, and SIGMA. "Alcohol Use and Unsafe Sexual Behaviour: Any Connection?" In *AIDS: Rights, Risks and Reason*, edited by Peter Aggleton, Peter Davies, and Graham Hart, 119–32. London: Falmer Press, 1992.

Westacott, Russell. "Crystal-Meth: Big Apple-Style." *HIV Australia* 5, no. 2 (2005): 17–19.

Westhaver, Russell. " 'Coming out of Your Skin': Circuit Parties, Pleasure and the Subject." *Sexualities* 8, no. 3 (2005): 347–74.

Wodak, Alex. "Taking Up Arms against a Sea of Drugs." *Meanjin* 61, no. 2 (2002): 44–58.

Worth, Heather, and Patrick Rawstorne. "Crystallizing the HIV Epidemic: Methamphetamine, Unsafe Sex, and Gay Diseases of the Will." *Archives of Sexual Behaviour* 34, no. 5 (2005): 483–86.

Young, Iris Marion. *Justice and the Politics of Difference*. Princeton: Princeton University Press, 1990.

Young, Jock. "The Myth of the Drug Taker in the Mass Media." In *The Manufacture of News*, edited by Stanley Cohen and Jock Young, 314–22. London: Constable, 1973.

Young, Katharine. "Disembodiment: The Phenomenology of the Body in Medical Examinations." *Semiotica* 73, no. 1–2 (1989): 43–66.

INDEX

...

Kane Race is a senior lecturer in gender and
cultural studies at the University of Sydney.

• • •

Library of Congress Cataloging-in-Publication Data
Race, Kane.
Pleasure consuming medicine : the queer politics
of drugs / Kane Race.
p. cm.
Includes bibliographical references and index.
ISBN 978-0-8223-4488-9 (cloth : alk. paper)
ISBN 978-0-8223-4501-5 (pbk. : alk. paper)
1. Drug abuse—Social aspects. 2. Pleasure.
3. Drugs and sex. 4. Gays—Drug use. I. Title.
HV5801.R29 2009
306'.1–dc22   2009003273